PALEO DIET FOR BEGINNERS

Get Healthy With Modern Paleo Diet Meal Plan

(Weekly Meal Plans and Recipes to Eat Healthy at Work)

Annette Vaden

Published by Alex Howard

Annette Vaden

All Rights Reserved

Paleo Diet for Beginners: Get Healthy With Modern Paleo Diet Meal Plan (Weekly Meal Plans and Recipes to Eat Healthy at Work)

ISBN 978-1-77485-024-4

All rights reserved. No part of this guide may be reproduced in any form without permission in writing from the publisher except in the case of brief quotations embodied in critical articles or reviews.

Legal & Disclaimer

The information contained in this book is not designed to replace or take the place of any form of medicine or professional medical advice. The information in this book has been provided for educational and entertainment purposes only.

The information contained in this book has been compiled from sources deemed reliable, and it is accurate to the best of the Author's knowledge; however, the Author cannot guarantee its accuracy and validity and cannot be held liable for any errors or omissions. Changes are periodically made to this book. You must consult your doctor or get professional medical advice before using any of the suggested remedies, techniques, or information in this book.

Upon using the information contained in this book, you agree to hold harmless the Author from and against any damages, costs, and expenses, including any legal fees potentially resulting from the application of any of the information provided by this guide. This disclaimer applies to any damages or injury caused by the use and application, whether directly or indirectly, of any advice or information presented, whether for breach of contract, tort, negligence, personal injury, criminal intent, or under any other cause of action.

You agree to accept all risks of using the information presented inside this book. You need to consult a professional medical practitioner in order to ensure you are both able and healthy enough to participate in this program.

Table of Contents

Part 1 1
Introduction 2
Chapter 1: Overview And Benefits Of Paleo Diet 3
Chapter 2: What To Eat And What To Avoid 7
Chapter 3: Advises For The Followers Of Paleo Diet 11
Chapter 4: 30 Day (4 Weeks) Meal Plan 13
Chapter 5: Paleo Breakfast Recipes 20
Recipe 01: Bacon And Egg Muffin 20
Recipe 02: Curry Omelet 22
Recipe 03: Mix Fruit Salad 24
Recipe 04: Baked Paleo Eggs In Avocado 25
Recipe 05: Fruit Salad With Lime And Honey 27
Recipe 06: Cauliflower Rice Paleo Frittata 28
Recipe 07: Breakfast Salsa 30
Chapter 6: Paleo Lunch Recipes 31
Recipe 08: Roasted Butternut Squash 31
Recipe 09: Brussels Sprouts 33
Recipe 10: Garlic And Roasted Tomato 34
Recipe 11: Crab Ceviche 35
Recipe 12: Mushroom Salad 36
Recipe 13: Cucumber Salad 37
Recipe 14: Almond And Bacon Salad 38
Recipe 15: Paleo Pizza Crust 40
Chapter 7: Paleo Dinner Recipes 41

Recipe 16: Salmon Cake 41

Recipe 17: Chicken With Coconut Milk 42

Recipe 18: Spinach Soup 44

Recipe 19: Beef Soup 46

Recipe 20: Gherkins Salad 47

Recipe 21: Shrimp Harissa 48

Recipe 22: Onion Soup 49

Chapter 8: Paleo Snacks And Dessert Recipes 51

Recipe 23: Cacao And Almond Bars 51

Recipe 24: Sorbet With Apple 52

Recipe 25: Stuffed Dates 53

Recipe 26: Delicious Macaroon 53

Recipe 27: Applesauce Cake Without Sugar 54

Recipe 28: Cornflakes Cookies 56

Recipe 29: Coconut Cookies 57

Recipe 30: Pancakes 58

Conclusion 60

Part 2 61

The Paleo Diet – An Introduction 62

The Paleo Diet - Covering The Basics 66

What Can Paleo Do For Me? 70

Studies 71

Can It Work For Diabetes? 71

Paleo Is Rich In Omega-3 72

Sugar – The Devil You Know 76

Dairy, Dairy Quite Contrary. 78

Would You Put Chip Pan Oil In Your Ferrari? 81

Legumes – Not What It Says On The Box. 83

History Of Paleo 84

So What Is The Paleo Diet Anyway? 85

The Crucial Do's And Don'ts 91

The Sensational Paleo Celebrities 97

7 Days Of Paleo Eating – Breakfast, Lunch, Dinner And Snack Recipes 104

Monday 107

Breakfast 107

Carrot Muffins 107

Lunch 108

Seafood Mint Salad 108

Dinner 109

Louisiana Fish 109

Snack 110

Zucchini Fries 111

Dessert 112

Chocolate Chip Cookies 112

Tuesday 113

Breakfast 113

Berry Pancakes 113

Lunch 114

Grilled Chicken Salad 114

Dinner 115

Shepherd's Pie 115

Snack 117

Veggie Fries	117
Dessert	118
Zesty Pudding	118
Wednesday	120
Breakfast	120
Tapioca Crepes	120
Lunch	121
Crab Bisque	121
Dinner	122
Beef Casserole	122
Snack	124
Trail Mix	124
Dessert	124
Butterscotch Ice Cream	124
Thursday	125
Breakfast	125
Vegetable Frittata	125
Lunch	127
Chicken Wraps	127
Dinner	128
Paleo Hamburgers	128
Snack	129
Blueberry Candy	129
Dessert	130
Creamy Flan	130
Friday	131

Breakfast 132

Western Omelet 132

Lunch 133

Burritos 133

Dinner 134

Snack 135

Chocolate Cake 135

Dessert 136

Grilled Bananas 137

Saturday 137

Breakfast 137

Lunch 139

Chicken Fajitas 139

Dinner 140

Snack 141

Salmon Poppers 141

Dessert 142

Almond Macaroons 142

Sunday 143

Breakfast 143

Pumpkin Muffins 144

Lunch 145

Grilled Veggies 145

Dinner 146

Vegetable And Turkey Meatballs 146

Snack 147

Deviled Eggs With Guacamole 147
Dessert 148
Brownies..148
What About Exercise?..150
Eating Out..164
Staying Motivated..173
Faq 175
Conclusion 184

Part 1

Introduction

Paleo diet is a healthy way to eat food and get rid of harmful effects of processed foods. The Paleo diet was first time introduced in the 1960s, but it was failed to get the attention of people. In 1975, people started noticing it because it is about food and eating habits of your ancestors. Following a Paleo diet doesn't mean to live in caves, hunt for food and live without modern amenities. It is all about food instead of a lifestyle and you can follow this diet to get lots of health benefits.

Some Paleo eaters are also allowed to consume fruits and nuts except peanuts because these fall in the category of legumes. You have to include raw and clean food in your diet while dumping grains, legumes, sugar, dairy and processed food. The omega-3 fats, olive oil, coconut oil and vegetable oils are allowed, but the refined oils are prohibited. You have to eat real food, such as the food that you can hunt and grow, despite starchy vegetables.

The Paleo diet is particularly designed to avoid the worst effects of overly-processed and carbohydrate food. The western diet is not good for your health because you may suffer from lots of chronic diseases. The type 2 diabetes, cancer and cardiovascular diseases are common with the consumption of processed food. The processed food promotes obesity and digestive issues and creates havoc in your life. The Paleo diet is a good step toward a healthy body because the real food will save you from lots of health problems.

This book is designed as a guide for you so that you can learn about Paleo diet, meal plans. And recipes. If you want to follow a Paleo diet, then this book will be a good start for you.

Chapter 1: Overview And Benefits Of Paleo Diet

The Paleolithic diet is simple and straightforward because it requires you to get rid of processed and high-carb food. You will follow the diet of a caveman while avoiding lectins and gluten. You need to eat natural food and avoid all types of processed and unhealthy food. High consumption of processed food, gluten and carbohydrates may lead you to obesity, cancer, diabetes and reproductive problems. People often misunderstand Paleo diet and try to avoid it, but, in fact, it is a beneficial diet. It is all about food because people often misunderstand that it means to follow a caveman lifestyle. You have to change your eating habits and stick to real food.

Benefits of Paleo Diet

The Paleo diet is a healthy way to eat and avoid lots of health problems. It can keep you lean, strong and energetic while reducing the threat of diabetes, heart diseases, cancer, obesity, and infertility. You have to avoid a modern diet that is full of refined foods, sugar and trans fats. There are some benefits of Paleo Diet that will help you to understand how this diet is good for your health:

Get Healthy Cells

The human body cells are made of saturated and unsaturated fat and the composition of your cell is based on a healthy diet. The paleo diet can naturally balance your body fat by limiting the consumption of unhealthy food. The Omega-3 fatty acids play an important role to enhance the performance of the brain and promote better growth and development.

Increase Muscle and Reduce Fat

Paleo diet is based on animal meat and it is a healthy source of protein. The anabolic protein is used to build new cells and it will increase your muscle mass. The more muscles will increase your metabolism rate and you will get more energy to move bigger muscles. It proves helpful for the body to send energy to muscle cells instead of fat cells. An increase in the muscle cells will automatically reduce the fat cells. The healthy paleo diet will help your body to increase the energy to transport to glycogen in your muscles instead of triglycerides found in fat cells. Muscles require more energy than fat and with a higher percentage of muscle than fat, you may have a higher BMR.

Better Gut Health

The sugar and processed food can increase your body fat and cause inflammation in your intestinal tract. The processed food can be the reason of stress because it may cause leaky gut syndrome. If you want to avoid problems with the digestive tract, then you should follow Paleo diet. The bolus of blood sugar with meals and refined carbohydrates, such as white bread, white rice, and sugar loaded soda can increase the levels of cytokines also known as an inflammatory messenger.

Circle of Life

The Paleo diet promotes the consumption of meats and eggs raised on pasture. The animals should be raised naturally on grass for their entire life. The cows and chickens should roam together in the meadow for better synergy. In the natural environment, the chickens eat larvae and bugs found under the cow pies. The cow pie can be a great fertilizer for the grass and it will provide food to the cows. The natural diet is great for animals because this food is loaded with nutrients and these animals will be healthy for your diet. The eggs and meat raised in a pasture contain 10 times more omega3s than the factory hens and eggs.

Lots of Vitamins and Minerals

You can eat a variety of vegetables and fruits of different colors. To get better health, it will be good to make your plate colorful by including a variety of vegetables and fruits of the season. The colors of the vegetables reflect the presence of particular nutrients. You can eat rainbow to get all your vitamins.

Limit Fructose

The human body reacts differently to digest fructose than other carbohydrates. The Paleo diet suggests the limited consumption of fructose; therefore, you have to be very careful while selecting fruit. You should avoid banana and include Kiwi in your diet. It is good to limit your diet to 2 to 3 pieces of fruit on a regular basis.

Digestion and Absorption

The paleo diet will increase your ability to digest and absorb food because the grass-fed beef is better than factory raised meat. A strict paleo diet for 30 days is good to solve your digestion problems. You will feel better after 30 days because the paleo diet can solve lots of digestion and absorption problems. Food items consumed in the paleo diet can help you to get rid of allergies and additional body fat.

Good for Allergies and Inflammation

The paleo diet will help you to reduce the consumption of allergens, such as grains. After reducing the consumption of grains, you can get rid of lots of allergies. It is good for inflammation and cardiovascular diseases because this diet focuses on Omega 3 fatty acids. The animals raised in the meadow have a better ratio of omega 3 and 6.

Better to Reduce Weight

The Paleo diet will help you to reduce weight and get more energy by reducing the consumption of sugar, coffee, and unhealthy fat. The paleo diet aka low carb diet is good for your health because after removing processed foods, you can drastically reduce additional pounds. You can increase your insulin sensitivity because sugary foods are not good for your health. It will reduce the risk of various diseases and shrink fat cells.

Chapter 2: What To Eat And What To Avoid

In order to follow a Paleo diet, you have to avoid consumption of particular food items. You should be careful with the food that you can eat or avoid:

If you want to follow a paleo meal, it is important to have all relevant ingredients in your pantry. You need to buy whole foods and it will be better to visit the farmer's market for the fresh fruits, vegetables, meats and other important items.

Buy Lean Meats

There are 10 essential animal proteins that should be unprocessed and free from hormone and antibiotic. The animals should be naturally raised in the meadow:

- Beef, Bison, and Buffalo

- Chicken, Turkey, and Duck (Free from skin and fat)

- Eggs

- Game Meats (Venison, Rabbit, Wild Boar)

- Lamb and Goat

- Kidneys, sweetbreads, tongue, livers and marrow organs

Sea Food

You can buy Paleo-friendly seafood because it has lots of protein and Omega fats to promote weight loss:

- Cod

- Anchovies

- Flounder
- Bass
- Halibut
- Salmon
- Mahi Mahi
- Shellfish (mussels, shrimp, crab, lobster and scallops)
- Sardines
- Tuna

Paleo Fruits

There are lots of fruits that are allowed in the Paleo diet, but you should avoid high sugar food. There are some simple guidelines for the selection of fruits in the Paleo diet

Limit the Consumption of High-sugar Fruits

Your diet should not include banana, mangoes, pineapple, dates and watermelon. You should avoid them if you are trying to reduce weight.

Dried Fruits

You can consume moderate amounts of dried fruits; such as mix one spoon in the salad to use as snacks. The nuts should be free from excessive sugar and salt because these can increase your calorie intake. You should consume in moderation because high consumption of dried fruit is not good for your health.

Avocados are Important

The Avocados have the healthy fats and you should include them in your diet.

Paleo Vegetables

Just like fruits, you can consume almost every vegetable, but be careful with starchy tubers. There are two notable things about the shopping of vegetables:

- Starchy Tubers: You should limit the consumption of potatoes and sweet potatoes because their excessive amounts are not good.
- Legumes: Chickpeas, peas, soybeans, and lentils are not good to take in Paleo diet because you should remove them from your list.

Nuts and Seeds

Nuts and seeds are famous for using as snacks in the paleo diet and these are great to give a crunchy touch to your recipes. Make sure to have them without any added salt, sugar, and unhealthy fat. You are not allowed to take peanuts because these are also considered a form of legume.

- Good Nuts for Paleo Diet: Cashews, Almonds, Macadamia Nuts, Walnuts, Pecans, Pistachios, etc.
- Good Seeds for Paleo Diet: Pumpkin, Sunflower, Sesame, Flaxseeds

Healthy Oils

Healthy oils are important for health, but in Paleo diet, you can't use vegetable oil, canola and peanut oil. Highly refined oils are not good for your health because these have a high concentration of polyunsaturated omega 6 fatty acids that can be the reason of inflammation in your body. You need oil with high omega-3 that can reduce inflammation. Try to buy paleo approved oils that are available in the most unprocessed form, such as extra-virgin olive oil.

- To use as salad dressings, you can use avocado oil. It is also good to cook food on a low heat.

- Coconut oil is good for all kinds of cooking.

- Flaxseed oils are excellent to use as omega 3 supplements.

- Extra-virgin olive oil is good to use in salad, cooking, and frying.

- Sesame oil will be seasoned on the cooked food.

- You can use small amounts of walnut oil in salads.

Healthy Beverages

If you want to include healthy beverages in your diet, then pick fresh juices and flavored milk without high sugar concentration. You can the following beverages:

- Coffee and tea without sugar and milk

- Soda water

- Coconut water

- Almond milk

- Plain Water

- Coconut milk

Sweets and Treats for Paleo Diet

You can take a limited amount of alcohol in the Paleo diet, but make it an occasional treat only. The dark chocolate is good for your heart and you can add unprocessed honey to your meals to make them sweet. Coconut products and stevia are also good to take as zero calorie sweeteners.

Chapter 3: Advises For The Followers Of Paleo Diet

There are some tips that will help you to build a healthy paleo diet because there are some foods that should be included in your diet:

Lean Proteins

Lean proteins are important for strong muscles, healthy bones, and best possible immune function. The protein will increase your satisfaction level and reduce your craving for unhealthy foods.

Fruits and Vegetables

The fruits and vegetables are good for your health because these are rich in vitamins, mineral, antioxidants and phytonutrients. Consumption of fruits and vegetables can decrease the chances diabetes, cancer, and neurological problems.

Healthy Fats

You should consume healthy fat obtained from nuts, avocados, seeds, fish oil, olive and grass-fed meat. The Omega-3 and monounsaturated fats will help you to reduce the chances of cancer, diabetes, cardiovascular disease and obesity.

Paleo Diet Routine

The Paleo diet is based on the unprocessed foods because this diet is good to avoid obesity, diabetes, and cardiovascular diseases. There is no right way to eat food, but you have to focus on the healthy foods and avoid dairy, grains, legumes, soybean, sunflower, corn and grape seed oil. There is a sample diet routine that will help you to follow a paleo diet:

Paleo Breakfast

At the breakfast, you can make an omelet with broccoli, mushrooms, and onion. Make sure to use olive oil, omega-3 enriched food and slices of chicken breast.

Paleo Lunches

In the initial week, you can enjoy a salad with mixed greens, radishes, spinach, bell peppers, carrots, cucumber, almonds, avocados, walnuts, apples, pears, etc. The salads can be prepared with the combination of different vegetables, nuts, and fruits. You can use olive oil and black pepper to enhance the flavor or your salad. Lemon juice is important to reduce body fat. You can mix pieces of chicken, beef, turkey or lamb. Seafood is a good choice, such as salmon, tuna, seafood, etc.

Paleo Dinner

In the dinner, you can try spaghetti squash with pasta that should be topped with marinara and pesto. Roasted beet and chicken will be a great dinner with steamed broccoli, spinach, and steamed asparagus. Salmon, tuna, and halibut are great to grill with olive oil and garlic. Your dinner should be packed with vegetables and lean meat to get lots of proteins.

Paleo Desserts

You can get the advantage of berries and other succulent fruits because it is great for dessert. The carrot, celery stick and slices of fruits are great to satisfy your dessert cravings.

Chapter 4: 30 Day (4 Weeks) Meal Plan

If you want to reduce weight, you can get the advantage of a 30-day diet plan. This sample diet plan has simple and easy recipes, but you can change these recipes with healthy paleo recipes:

Day 01

Breakfast: Kale Frittata

Lunch: Tomato Zucchini Salad

Dinner: Paleo Orange Chicken

Day 02

Breakfast: **Baked Eggs**

Lunch: Kale and Carrot Salad

Dinner: Salmon with walnut and cucumber

Day 03

Breakfast: Baked Eggs and Mushrooms

Lunch: Paleo Salad

Dinner: Chicken breast

Day 04

Breakfast: Has Browns Eggs

Lunch: Fruit Salad and Coconut Cream

Dinner: Kale and Root Veggies

Day 05

Breakfast: Egg Muffins

Lunch: **Enchiladas**

Dinner: Curry Shrimp

Day 06

Breakfast: Kale Smoothie

Lunch: Roasted Chicken

Dinner: Brussels Sprouts with Almond and Bacon

Day 07

Breakfast: Cocoa Nibs, Kefir and Hemp Seeds

Lunch: Chicken and Greens Salad

Dinner: Turkey or Chicken Burgers

Day 08

Breakfast: Eggs and Bacon

Lunch: Avocado and watermelon salad

Dinner: Tuna Petties

Day 09

Breakfast: Blueberry Muffins

Lunch: Zucchini Noodles with Tomato Sauce

Dinner: Spaghetti Squash, Chicken and Mushrooms

Day 10

Breakfast: Scrambled Eggs and Avocado

Lunch: Tuna Salad

Dinner: Almond Chicken

Day 11

Breakfast: Cinnamon Waffles

Lunch: Avocado and Broccoli Salad

Dinner: **Lasagna**

Day 12

Breakfast: Coconut pancake

Lunch: Summer Salad

Dinner: Stir fry chicken

Day 13

Breakfast: Chocolate Pancakes

Lunch: Chicken Salad

Dinner: Paleo Pie

Day 14

Breakfast: Lemon Pancakes

Lunch: Egg Salad

Dinner: Salmon with Mushroom and Leek

Day 15

Breakfast: Coconut Smoothie

Lunch: Avocado, kale and orange salad

Dinner: Zucchini Beef

Day 16

Breakfast: Scrambled or hard-boiled eggs

Lunch: Avocado and asparagus salad

Dinner: Confetti Coleslaw

Day 17

Breakfast: Paleo veggie and chicken pizza

Lunch: Broccoli chick salad

Dinner: Kale and spiced turkey

Day 18

Breakfast: Paleo pancakes

Lunch: Arugula beet noodle salad

Dinner: Delicious steak

Day 19

Breakfast: Zucchini and pumpkin muffins

Lunch: Strawberry and lavender soup

Dinner: Curry chicken

Day 20:

Breakfast: Chocolate milkshake

Lunch: Raw vegetable salad

Dinner: Salmon with pumpkin and sweet potato

Day 21

Breakfast: Apple cinnamon banana shake

Lunch: Paleo turnip soup

Dinner: Vegetable and chicken kebabs

Day 22

Breakfast: Egg salad with lettuce

Lunch: Roasted beef with vegetables

Dinner: Plantain chips

Day 23

Breakfast: Roasted beef with pesto

Lunch: Cabbage poach and beef

Dinner: Mustard pork with coleslaw

Day 24

Breakfast: Egg with salsa

Lunch: Coconut curry

Dinner: Cauliflower and smoked tuna

Day 25

Breakfast: Fried beef and carrot

Lunch: Boiled eggs and bacon with tomato

Dinner: Stew and pumpkin seed

Day 26

Breakfast: Asparagus and chicken omelet

Lunch: Garlic sauce and mussels

Dinner: Chicken with lemon, garlic and olive

Day 27

Breakfast: Beef liver and baked broccoli

Lunch: Fried lamb chops and spinach

Dinner: Pumpkin chili

Day 28

Breakfast: Spinach and onion omelet

Lunch: Tuna salad with almonds and lettuce

Dinner: Squash soup and grilled trout

Day 29

Breakfast: Paleo spaghetti

Lunch: Vegetable and chicken soup

Dinner: Beef goulash

Day 30

Breakfast: Eggs and chicken with one fruit

Lunch: Sweet potato and zucchini

Dinner: Beef Bourguignon

Note: You can use fresh fruits and vegetables with healthy dip as snacks. It will help you to suppress your hunger.

Chapter 5: Paleo Breakfast Recipes

Start your day with a healthy breakfast, and here are some delicious recipes to make your morning work easy.

Recipe 01: Bacon And Egg Muffin

Total Time: 30 minutes

Servings: 6

Ingredients

 Filling

- ☐ Black pepper (ground): 1 pinch
- ☐ Eggs: 8
- ☐ Chopped green onion: 2 tablespoons
- ☐ Bacon: 6 slices
- ☐ Cooking spray: as per need
- ☐ Cherry tomatoes: 1 cup (halved)

Directions:

1. Preheat your oven to almost 350 °F. Spray nearly 6 muffin pans/cups with your cooking spray.

2. Put bacon in one large skillet and cook over medium heat. Turn occasionally, until halfway done, almost 5 minutes.

3. Blot all bacon slices with your paper towels and cut it into small slices.

4. Mix black pepper, green onion, tomatoes, eggs and bacon in one bowl. Pour this mixture into the greased muffin cups.

5. Bake in your preheated oven for almost 15 – 20 minutes, until the muffins set in the center.

Recipe 02: Curry Omelet

Total Time: 30 minutes

Servings: 1

Ingredients

Filling

- ☐ Light sesame oil: 1 tablespoon
- ☐ Minced garlic: 1/2 teaspoon
- ☐ Minced onion: 2 tablespoons
- ☐ Green onion (sliced): 2 tablespoons
- ☐ Diced bell pepper (red): 1/4 cup
- ☐ Salt: 1/4 teaspoon
- ☐ Ground coriander: 1/2 teaspoon
- ☐ Ground cumin: 1/2 teaspoon
- ☐ Ground turmeric: 1/2 teaspoon
- ☐ Beaten eggs: 2

Directions:

1. Heat some sesame oil in the skillet over medium flame. Mix in garlic and cook it for nearly 20 seconds to get fragrance.

2. Stir in salt, bell pepper, green onion and onion. Cook for almost one minute to make vegetables soft.

3. Sprinkle with turmeric, cumin and coriander and cook for nearly 30 seconds.

4. Equally spread vegetables on the base of your skillet. Pour in whisked eggs and gently cook to make it set, now turn over and cook for extra 30 seconds to make it firm.

5. Roll omelet on the plate to serve.

Recipe 03: Mix Fruit Salad

Total Time: 15 minutes

Servings: 4

Ingredients

Filling

- ☐ Golden raisins: ¼ cup
- ☐ Peeled and chopped oranges (bite sizes slices): 2
- ☐ Red grapes (seedless): 1 cup
- ☐ Chopped dates (pitted): ¼ cup
- ☐ Walnut halves: ¼ cup
- ☐ Halved and pitted cherries: ½ cup

Directions:

1. Combine the walnut, dates, raisins, cherries, grapes, and orange pieces in one bowl.

2. Toss well to combine and serve chilled.

Recipe 04: Baked Paleo Eggs In Avocado

Total Time: 25 minutes

Servings: 2

Ingredients

 Filling

- ☐ Small eggs: 2
- ☐ Chopped chives: 2 teaspoons
- ☐ Pitted and halved avocado: 1
- ☐ Dried parsley: 1 pinch
- ☐ Powdered black pepper and sea salt: as per taste
- ☐ Crumbled bacon: 2 slices

Directions:

1. Preheat your oven to almost 425 °F.

2. Crack all eggs in the bowl, but be careful to keep their yolks intact.

3. Arrange halves of avocado in one baking dish and rest them along their edges to avoid tipping over. Slowly spoon one egg yolk in the hole of avocado. Spoon egg white in the hole to make it full.

4. Replicate this procedure with remaining yolk, egg white and avocado. Season every avocado with pepper, sea salt, parsley and chives.

5. Slowly put baking dish in your preheated oven and bake eggs for almost 15 minutes. Sprinkle some bacon over baked avocado.

Recipe 05: Fruit Salad With Lime And Honey

Total Time: 20 minutes

Servings: 8

Ingredients

Filling

- ☐ Sliced bananas: 2 large
- ☐ Honey: 2 tablespoons
- ☐ Lime juice: Juice 1 lime
- ☐ Pine nuts: 1/3 cup
- ☐ Strawberries (sliced and hulled): 16 ounces
- ☐ Blueberries: ½ pound

Directions:

1. Combine blueberries, strawberries and bananas in one bowl. Drizzle some lime juice and honey over mixed fruits.

2. Stir well to coal all fruits and sprinkle with some pine nuts. Serve chilled.

Recipe 06: Cauliflower Rice Paleo Frittata

Total Time: 30 minutes

Servings: 4

Ingredients

Filling

- ☐ Cauliflower (broken in large pieces): 1 large cauliflower head
- ☐ Avocado oil: 2 tablespoons
- ☐ Garlic salt: 1 pinch
- ☐ Egg whites: 2 cups
- ☐ Eggs: 4
- ☐ Garlic powder: 1 pinch,
- ☐ Black pepper (ground): 1 pinch
- ☐ Red pepper flakes: 1 pinch

Directions:

1. Set your oven rack to almost 6-inches to a heat source and preheat the broiler of your oven.

2. Run the cauliflower pieces in your food processor with the use of shred blade to create rice.

3. Heat oil in the oven-safe skillet over medium heat. Add garlic salt and cauliflower rice and stir well for almost 3 – 4 minutes.

4. Whisk salt, black pepper, garlic powder, eggs and egg whites together in one bowl. Pour cauliflower mixture over egg white blend and cook well for almost 5 – 7 minutes.

5. Put the skillet under your broiler for almost 5 – 7 minutes to cook well. Let it cool for 5 minutes and serve.

Recipe 07: Breakfast Salsa

Total Time: 15 minutes

Servings: 6

Ingredients

Filling

- ☐ Bacon: 9 slices
- ☐ Chopped tomato: 1 fresh
- ☐ Chopped onion: ½
- ☐ Tomato sauce: ½ cup
- ☐ Jalapeno pepper (chopped and seeded): 1 fresh

Directions:

1. Put bacon in the deep and large skillet. Cook it over medium heat to make it equally brown.

2. Turn off heat and drain bacon on two paper towels. Pour some grease from your pan and leave one thin coating.

3. Sauté pepper, tomato and onions in one pan to make onion soft, for almost 3 minutes. Crumble cooked slices of back in the pan and stir in delicious tomato sauce. Cook constantly to heat through.

4. Serve hot with coconut tortilla.

Chapter 6: Paleo Lunch Recipes

Paleo lunch is really important to deal with your craving. It is important to have something healthy. Here are a few recipes to enjoy pale lunch.

Recipe 08: Roasted Butternut Squash

Total Time: 15 minutes

Servings: 4

Ingredients

Filling

- ☐ Chopped bacon: 4 slices
- ☐ Red pepper flakes: 1 teaspoon
- ☐ Minced garlic: 1 teaspoon
- ☐ Bok choy: 2 pounds
- ☐ Olive oil: 1 teaspoon
- ☐ Salt: as per taste
- ☐ Chopped red onion: ½ small

Directions:

1. Fry bacon slices in one large pan over medium flame to make them crispy. Remove fried bacon and drain their fat. Reserve almost one tablespoon of grease in your skillet.

2. Add garlic, red pepper flakes, onion and olive oil in the pan. Cook well over medium heat to tender onion.

3. Now add bok choy in the pan and cover this pan with a lid. Cook it for 3 – 5 minutes. Remove lid and stir well for almost 2 minutes to tender bok choy.

4. Mix in bacon and season with some pepper and salt. Serve hot.

Recipe 09: Brussels Sprouts

Total Time: 30 minutes

Servings: 4

Ingredients

Filling

- ☐ Water: 3 cups
- ☐ Diced pancetta bacon: 8 ounces
- ☐ Salt: 1 teaspoon
- ☐ Trimmed Brussels sprouts: 1 pound
- ☐ Black pepper (ground): 1 teaspoon
- ☐ Olive oil: 2 tablespoons
- ☐ Minced garlic: 2 cloves

Directions:

1. Boil water in a saucepan and add all Brussels sprouts to cook for 5 – 7 minutes. Keep them slightly firm. Drain them and rinse with cool water. Make slices of Brussels sprouts in half and keep them aside.

2. Heat 1 tablespoons olive oil in one large pan over medium flame. Add pancetta and garlic and cook for almost 5 minutes to make garlic brown.

3. Add the Brussels sprouts and remaining olive oil. Decrease heat to cook on medium flame and stir sprouts well to coat them with all flavors. Season with pepper and salt and cook for five minutes. Serve hot.

Recipe 10: Garlic And Roasted Tomato

Total Time: 25 minutes

Servings: 6

Ingredients

Filling

- ☐ Olive oil: 2 tablespoons
- ☐ Grape tomatoes: 4 cups
- ☐ Pepper and salt: as per taste
- ☐ Sliced garlic: 4 cloves

Directions:

1. Preheat your oven to almost 450 °F. Line your baking dish with pieces of aluminum foil.

2. Put garlic and tomatoes in one mixing bowl. Drizzle with some olive oil and toss well to coat. Season with pepper and salt to taste.

3. Spread tomatoes equally on greased baking sheet. Bake these tomatoes in one preheated oven for almost 15 – 20 minutes.

4. Serve hot.

Recipe 11: Crab Ceviche

Total Time: 30 minutes

Servings: 8

Ingredients

Filling

- ☐ Imitation Crabmeat (flaked): 8 ounces
- ☐ Lime juice: squeeze 2 limes
- ☐ Chopped serrano peppers: 3
- ☐ Chopped tomatoes: 2 large
- ☐ Olive oil: 1 tablespoon
- ☐ Chopped red onion: 1
- ☐ Pepper and salt: as per taste
- ☐ Chopped cilantro: 1 bunch

Directions:

1. Put tattered imitation crab in one porcelain or glass bowl. Metal or plastic bowls are not recommended.

2. Mix olive oil in the crabmeat to coat well and mix in serrano peppers, tomato, onion and cilantro.

3. Squeeze both limes over everything and mix lime juice well.

4. Season with pepper and salt as per taste. put in the fridge for almost an hour before serving it.

Recipe 12: Mushroom Salad

Total Time: 25 minutes

Servings: 4

Ingredients

Filling

- ☐ Balsamic vinegar: 2 ½ tablespoons
- ☐ Olive oil: 1 tablespoon
- ☐ Pepper and salt: as per taste
- ☐ Fresh mushrooms (sliced): 1 ½ cups
- ☐ Chopped garlic: 1 clove
- ☐ Baby greens (mix): 10 ounces
- ☐ Olive oil: 2 ½ tablespoons

Directions:

1. Heat one tablespoon oil in one skillet over medium flame. Add fresh mushrooms and cook well until soft. Continue cook to reduce juices of mushrooms to almost 2 tablespoons

2. Mix in remaining olive oil, pepper, salt, and balsamic vinegar to make an even blend. Turn off flame and leave the mushrooms in pan so that they become just warm instead of hot.

3. Now put greens in one serving bowl and top with warm mushroom blend (hot mushrooms can excessively wilt greens). Mix this blend and serve.

Recipe 13: Cucumber Salad

Total Time: 20 minutes

Servings: 4

Ingredients

Filling

- ☐ Cider vinegar: ¼ cup
- ☐ Halved grape tomatoes: 1 pint
- ☐ Seeded and chopped cucumber: 3
- ☐ Olive oil: ¼ cup
- ☐ Chopped onion: 1
- ☐ Drained capers: 4 ounces
- ☐ Dried chill: 2 teaspoons
- ☐ Chopped bell pepper (yellow): 2

Directions:

1. Mix red onion, cucumbers, bell peppers and tomatoes in one bowl. Mix some olive oil vinegar, dill and capers.

2. Toss everything well to coat all ingredients. Serve chilled or at room temperature.

Recipe 14: Almond And Bacon Salad

Total Time: 35 minutes

Servings: 8

Ingredients

Filling

- ☐ Bacon: ½ pound
- ☐ Olive oil: ¼ cup
- ☐ White vinegar: 2 tablespoons
- ☐ Red lettuce (bite-size pieces): 1 head
- ☐ Mandarin oranges (drained): 15 ounces
- ☐ Honey: 3 tablespoons
- ☐ Diced green onion: 1 bunch
- ☐ Hot mustard (dry): ½ teaspoon
- ☐ Silvered almonds: ¾ cup
- ☐ Celery salt: ½ teaspoon
- ☐ Ground paprika: ½ teaspoon

Directions:

1. Take one medium skillet and put it over medium heat. Cook bacon to in the skillet to make it equally brown. Drain, let them cool and crumble bacon.

2. Now make dressing by mixing olive oil, paprika, celery salt, dry mustard, honey and vinegar in one bowl.

3. Now put almonds, bacon, green onion, oranges and lettuce in one serving bowl. Pour in dressing and mix all ingredients. Serve it warm or chilled.

Recipe 15: Paleo Pizza Crust

Total Time: 30 minutes

Servings: 4

Ingredients

Filling

- ☐ Coconut oil: 1 tablespoon
- ☐ Almond flour: 1 cup
- ☐ Flax seeds: 2 tablespoons
  - ☐ Egg: 1

Directions:

Preheat your oven to almost 350 °F. Cover the baking sheet with a parchment paper.

Blend flax seeds, coconut oil, egg, and almond flour in one blender. Transfer the blend to greased baking sheet and pressure or roll out to desired shape and thickness.

Top with desired toppings, such as vegetables, onion, olives, chicken slices and tomato ketchup.

Bake in the preheated oven to make it golden brown for almost 20 minutes.

Chapter 7: Paleo Dinner Recipes

There are a few delicious recipes to prepare dinner. These dinners are healthy for everyone to lose weight.

Recipe 16: Salmon Cake

Total Time: 30 minutes

Servings: 4

Ingredients

Filling

- ☐ Salmon (flaked and drained): 14.75 ounces
- ☐ Black pepper (ground): 1 teaspoon
- ☐ Whisked eggs: 2
- ☐ Vegetable oil: 3 tablespoons
- ☐ Diced onion: 1 small

Directions:

1. Remove all bones of salmon and separate all meat. Keep it aside.

2. Take one mixing bowl and whisk eggs in this bowl. Add pepper, salmon and diced onion in the bowl. Mix well.

3. Shape in two ounce patties (make almost 7 – 8 patties. Put one large skillet over medium flame and heat some oil. Fry every patty for almost 5 minutes on every side to make them golden brown and crispy.

Recipe 17: Chicken With Coconut Milk

Total Time: 30 minutes

Servings: 4

Ingredients

Filling

- ☐ Ground cumin: 1 teaspoon
- ☐ Chopped onion: 1
- ☐ Minced ginger: 1 tablespoon
- ☐ Cayenne pepper (ground): 1 teaspoon
- ☐ Chopped and seeded jalapeno peppers: 2
- ☐ Ground turmeric: 1 teaspoon
- ☐ Minced garlic: 2 cloves
- ☐ Ground coriander: 1 teaspoon
- ☐ Chopped and seeded tomatoes: 3
- ☐ Boneless and skinless chicken: 4 breast (halves)
- ☐ Coconut milk: 14 ounces
- ☐ Pepper and salt: as per taste
- ☐ Chopped parsley: 1 bunch
- ☐ Olive oil: 2 tablespoons

Directions:

1. Take one medium bowl and mix coriander, turmeric, cayenne pepper, and cumin in this bowl. Put chicken in the bowl

and season with pepper and salt as per taste. Rub all sides of chicken with the spice blends.

2.   Heat olive oil (1 tablespoon) in one skillet over medium flame. Put the chicken in skillet and cook every side for almost 10 – 15 minutes to make it light brown and clear all juices. Turn off heat and put it aside.

3.   Add remaining oil in the pan and heat it. Add garlic, jalapeno peppers, ginger and onion in the pan and cook for 5 minutes to tender.

4.   Stir in tomatoes and keep cooking for 5 – 8 minutes. Mix in coconut milk and serve it over cooked chicken. Garnish with some parsley.

Recipe 18: Spinach Soup

Total Time: 30 minutes

Servings: 8

Ingredients

Filling

- ☐ Olive oil: 3 tablespoons
- ☐ Ground allspice: ¼ teaspoon
- ☐ Chopped onion: 1
- ☐ Ground nutmeg: ¼ teaspoon
- ☐ Peeled & diced potatoes: 2
- ☐ Chopped celery: 2 stalks
- ☐ Chopped zucchini: 4 cups
- ☐ Minced garlic: 4 cloves
- ☐ Vegetable stock: 6 cups
- ☐ Minced ginger root: 2 tablespoons
- ☐ Cayenne pepper: 1 pinch
- ☐ Turbinado sugar: 1 tablespoons
- ☐ Chopped spinach: 1 cup
- ☐ Sea salt: 2 teaspoons
- ☐ Minced bell pepper (red): ½
- ☐ Ground turmeric: ¼ teaspoon

Directions:

Heat oil in one large pot or skillet over medium flame. Stir in sugar, ginger, garlic, celery and onion and cook them for five minutes to tender onion. Season with nutmeg, allspice, turmeric, and salt.

Add in zucchini and potatoes and stir in vegetable stock. Let this mixture boil and decrease heat to almost low and simmer for ten minutes to tender potatoes.

Turn off heat and season soup with cayenne pepper. Now mix in spinach and use one hand blender to blend this mixture and make it smooth. Garnish with some red bell pepper and serve warm.

Recipe 19: Beef Soup

Cooking time: 30 minutes

Servings: 2 to 3

Ingredients

Filling

- ☐ Dashi stock – 1 cup
- ☐ Soy sauce – ¾ cup
- ☐ Mirin – ¾ cup
- ☐ White sugar – ¼ cup
- ☐ Shirataki noodles – 8 oz.
- ☐ Canola oil – 2 tbsp.
- ☐ Sirloin beef (sliced) – 1 pound
- ☐ Onion (sliced) – 1
- ☐ Canola oil – 1 tbsp.
- ☐ Celery (sliced) – 2 stalks
- ☐ Carrots (sliced) – 2
- ☐ Green onions (pieces) – 5
- ☐ Mushrooms (sliced) – 4
- ☐ Tofu (cubes) – 14 oz.

Directions:

1. Get a bowl and mix the following ingredients together such as sugar, soy sauce, and mirin and dashi stock.

2. Take a pot and boil the noodles for 2 minutes. Make sure you keep a check on it and then take it off to rinse with cold water.
3. Now get a pan and heat it with adding canola oil in it. Cook the beef in it for about 10 minutes until it is soft and tender.
4. When the beef is cooked, add celery, mushrooms, carrot and onion in it. Stir it well so all mix well. Now add the green onions along with the noodles, tofu and dashi mixture.
5. Now when the entire mixture simmers, then serve it in a big bowl to enjoy it with your family!

Recipe 20: Gherkins Salad

Cooking Time: 25 minutes

Servings: 4

Ingredients

Filling

- ☐ Eggs: 8
- ☐ Brown mustard: ¼ teaspoon
- ☐ Dry mustard: ¼ teaspoon
- ☐ Mayonnaise: ½ cup
- ☐ Black pepper (ground) and salt: as per taste
- ☐ Green onion (chopped): 2 tablespoons
- ☐ Chopped celery: 2 tablespoons
- ☐ Paprika: ¼ teaspoon
- ☐ Chopped gherkins: 1 tablespoon

Directions:

1. In the first step, put eggs in one saucepan (in one layer) and cover all eggs with cold water. Place this pan on medium heat to let this water boil and decrease flame to low.

2. Cook eggs at low temperature for almost ten minutes. Turn off heat and drain hot water. Leave these boiled eggs under a running stream of water for a few moments to let them cool. Shell and chop eggs.

3. Stir dry mustard, brown mustard, gherkins, celery, green onion, mayonnaise and chopped eggs in a big bowl. Sprinkle pepper, salt and paprika over eggs and serve with crackers or fill in hollow tomato to serve.

Recipe 21: Shrimp Harissa

Cooking Time: 20 minutes

Servings: 2

Ingredients

Filling

- ☐ Frozen Shrimp: 30 to 40
- ☐ Water: ½ cup
- ☐ Spice mix (Ras el hanout): 1 tablespoon
- ☐ Chopped yellow onion: 1/3 cup
- ☐ Minced Garlic: 1 tablespoon
- ☐ Sea Salt: ½ teaspoon
- ☐ Chopped parsley (fresh): 1 tablespoon

- ☐ Chopped cilantro (fresh): 1 tablespoon
- ☐ Harissa sauce: 7 oz.
- ☐ Olive oil: 2 tablespoons
- ☐ Couscous (Cooked): 2 cups

Directions:

1. Preheat one oven to almost 400°F.

2. Wash shrimps with fresh water and let them boil in a pot filled with water for approximately 7 minutes on medium heat. Drain water and let them cool. Remove all shells on shrimps.

3. Put cooked prawns in one tagine bowl and add water, onion, mixed spice, salt, garlic, cilantro and parsley in this bowl. Now pour simmer sauce over the top and drizzle with some olive oil. Mix them well.

4. Keep this bowl in oven for almost 20 minutes without covering this bowl and in the meantime, use a stovetop to cook your couscous.

5. Take out this bowl from oven and put a tagine lid (cone-shaped) over to cover. Steam it for almost 5 to 10 minutes. Serve couscous and shrimp on a dish.

Recipe 22: Onion Soup

Cooking time: 30 minutes

Servings: 4

Ingredients

Filling

- ☐ Celery (chopped) – ½ stalk

- ☐ Onion (chopped) – 1
- ☐ Carrot (chopped) – ½
- ☐ Ginger (grated) – 1 tsp.
- ☐ Garlic (minced) – ½ tsp.
- ☐ Chicken stock – 2 tbsp.
- ☐ Bouillon beef granules - 3 tsp.
- ☐ Mushrooms (chopped) – 1 cup
- ☐ Water – 2 cups
- ☐ Baby mushrooms (sliced) – 1 cup
- ☐ Chives (chopped) – 1 tbsp.

Directions:

1. Get a pot and add the following ingredients to it such as onion, ginger, carrot, garlic, celery and mushrooms. Mix it well and then adds the chicken stock. Stir the entire mixture and let it cook for 5 minutes.

2. When it comes to a boil, then add the beef bouillon along with water in it. Now cover the lid and let it cook for 10 minutes.

3. Now place the remaining mushrooms on the bottom of a bowl and when the mixture of soup is ready, then pour it over in the bowl. It will mix all the ingredients along with the baby mushrooms.

4. Sprinkle the chives over the bowl and serve when ready!

Chapter 8: Paleo Snacks And Dessert Recipes

Satisfy your sweet tooth and satisfy your hunger between meals, you can get the advantage of these recipes.

Recipe 23: Cacao And Almond Bars

Servings: 1 bar

Preparation Time: 30 minutes

Ingredients

Filling

- ☐ Almonds: ¼ cup
- ☐ Cacao Nibs: ¼ cup
- ☐ Figs: 3
- ☐ Cacao Powder: 1 tablespoon
- ☐ Goji Berries: ¼ cup

Directions:

1. Add almonds in the short cup of blender to grind them with the help of pulsing techniques to get a chunky consistency.

2. Put crushed almonds in one bowl and scoop out the whole meat of rips figs and put in the bowl with almonds. Add in goji berries, cacao nibs, and cacao powder.

3. Mix all these ingredients well and take handfuls of this mixture and make a rectangular bar. You can wrap each bar in a wax paper. You can shape the mixture once again after wrapping it in the wax paper.

Recipe 24: Sorbet With Apple

Cooking Time: 30 minutes

Cooling Time: 4 hours 5 minutes

Servings: 8

Ingredients

Filling

- ☐ Smith apples (cored and sliced): 1 ¼ pounds
- ☐ Lemon juice: squeeze 1 ½ lemons
- ☐ Honey: 1 tablespoon
- ☐ Water: 1 ½ cups
- ☐ Sugar: 1 ½ cups

Directions:

Take a plastic container or resealable bag made of plastic and mix apples with lemon juice (1/2 juice) and freeze it for one night for a few hours.

Take one small saucepan and bring sugar and water to boil on medium heat. Decrease heat and simmer for almost five minutes. Turn off heat and mix in honey. Let this mixture cool completely.

Put the apple in the blender and liquidize these apples with remaining lemon juice and sugar syrup. Blend this mixture to make it smooth. Apple peels will give a unique texture to your sorbet.

You can transfer this blend to your ice cream machine and freeze it as per directions. Leave sorbet out for almost ten minutes before serving.

Recipe 25: Stuffed Dates

Cooking Time: 30 minutes

Servings: 25

Ingredients

Filling

- [ ] Chopped chocolate: 8 ounces
- [ ] Medjool dates (pitted): 25
- [ ] Pecan halves: 25
- [ ] Shredded coconut (sweetened): 2 tablespoons

Directions:

☐Put chocolate in a plastic or glass bowl and heat in your microwave for almost two minutes and stir after every thirty seconds to make it smooth.

☐Line your baking sheet with one aluminum foil and stuff every date with a pecan half and put on the baking sheet.

☐Drizzle melted chocolate on dates and sprinkle coconut over dates. Put these dates in the freezer and freeze for almost one hour. Serve with additional nuts as per your taste.

Recipe 26: Delicious Macaroon

Servings: 18

Total Time: 30 minutes

Ingredients

Filling

- ☐ Olive oil spray
- ☐ Flaked coconut (unsweetened): 2 1/2 cups
- ☐ Unbleached flour: 1 cup
- ☐ Cashews: 3/4 cup
- ☐ Water: 3/4 cup
- ☐ Raw sugar (Turbinado): 1/2 cup
- ☐ Salt: 1/2 teaspoon
- ☐ Almond extract: 1/2 teaspoon

Directions:

1. Preheat your oven to almost 350 °F. Grease baking sheet with your cooking spray.
2. Combine flour and coconut in one large bowl.
3. Use a blender to puree almond extract, salt, sugar, water and cashews. Stir cashew blend into coconut blend and mix them well.
4. Make 1-inch balls from coconut blend and make these balls flat. Arrange these balls on greased baking sheet.
5. Bake cookies in your preheated oven for almost 12 – 15 minutes to make edges golden.

Recipe 27: Applesauce Cake Without Sugar

Cooking Time: 30 minutes

Servings: 12

Ingredients

Filling

- ☐ Baking powder: 1 teaspoon
- ☐ Baking soda: 1 teaspoon
- ☐ Brown sugar or sugar substitute: ¾ cup
- ☐ Eggs: 2
- ☐ Vanilla extract: 1 teaspoon
- ☐ Ground cinnamon: ½ teaspoon
- ☐ Nutmeg (ground): ½ teaspoon
- ☐ Raisins: ½ cup
- ☐ Salt: ½ teaspoon
- ☐ All-purpose flour: 2 cups
- ☐ Unsweetened applesauce: 1 ½ cups

Directions:

1. Preheat an oven to almost 350 degrees F and grease one loaf pan with non-stick cooking spray. Keep it aside.

2. Sift baking powder, baking soda, cinnamon, salt, nutmeg, and flour together. Keep it aside.

3. Beat all eggs and mix in sugar, vanilla, and applesauce. Add a mixture of flour in the egg mixture and beat well to make them smooth. It is time to add raisins.

4. Pour this batter into greased loaf pan and bake in your preheated oven for almost one hour. Insert a toothpick in the middle, if it comes out clean, your cake is ready. Serve chilled.

Recipe 28: Cornflakes Cookies

Servings: 24

Total Time: 30 minutes

Ingredients

Filling

- ☐ Brown sugar (packed): 1 cup
- ☐ Diet sugar: 1/2 cup
- ☐ Softened butter: 1/2 cup
- ☐ Vanilla extract: 1 teaspoon
- ☐ Eggs: 2
- ☐ All-purpose flour: 3/4 cup
- ☐ Cornflakes cereal: 5 cups
- ☐ Flaked coconut: 1 1/2 cups

Directions:

1. Preheat your oven to almost 375 °F. Line your cookie sheets with dual parchment paper.

2. Cream white sugars, brown sugar, and butter in a bowl and add vanilla and eggs in this mixture. Whisk well.

3. Stir in flour and mix well to combine. Mix in coconut and corn flakes. Blend this mixture well and drop on a baking sheet lined with parchment paper by teaspoonfuls.

4. Bake in your preheated oven for almost 8 – 10 minutes.

Recipe 29: Coconut Cookies

Servings: 8

Total Time: 30 minutes

Ingredients

Filling

- ☐ Egg whites: 2 large
- ☐ White sugar: 1/2 cup
- ☐ Salt: 1/8 teaspoon
- ☐ Lime juice: 1 teaspoon
- ☐ Toasted and flake coconut: 7 ounces
- ☐ Cocoa powder (unsweetened): 1 tablespoon

Directions:

1. Preheat your oven to almost 300 °F. Line your cookie sheets with dual parchment paper.

2. Whisk egg whites until foamy in on metal or glass mixing bowl. Slowly add sugar and continue whisking to make soft peaks.

3. Now lift your beater or beat straight up. Egg whites may make soft mounds instead of sharp peaks. Add lime juice and salt and continue whisking until you notice a sharp peak that

manages its shape as you stop whisking. Gently mix the cocoa powder and coconut in this mixture.

4. Drop this mixture via tablespoonfuls on lined baking sheets. Bake for almost 20 minutes to make this mixture golden brown. Cool on pans and transfer to your wire racks. Store in one airtight container for later use.

Recipe 30: Pancakes

Cooking Time: 20 minutes

Servings: 4

Ingredients:

Pancakes

- ☐ Coconut Flour: 1 cup
- ☐ Coconut (low-fat): 1 cup
- ☐ Almond milk: ¼ cup
- ☐ One pinch salt

Topping

- ☐ Chopped apples: 1 cup
- ☐ Cinnamon powder: ¼ teaspoon
- ☐ Sugar Substitute: 1 tablespoon or as per taste

Procedure:

Apple Topping

Combine ¼ cup water and apple in one pan and let them boil. Simmer for almost 5 – 7 minutes to let the apples soft. Add sugar substitute and cinnamon powder in apples and mix them well.

Pancakes

Mix all ingredients of pancakes in a bowl and whisk them together to make a smooth batter. Leave it for almost ten minutes. Pour one-quarter of low-fat butter on a non-stick pan.

Pour some batter into the pan and spread this mixture. Let it cook to make one side golden and then flip its side. Once both sides turn golden brown, transfer pancake to a plate. Make as many pancakes as you can and serve them with apple topping.

Note: You can make buttermilk by whisking some water and five tablespoons of curds.

Conclusion

The Paleo diet is particularly designed to avoid the worst effects of overly-processed and carbohydrate food. The western diet is not good for your health because you may suffer from lots of chronic diseases.

The type 2 diabetes, cancer and cardiovascular diseases are common with the consumption of processed food. The processed food promotes obesity and digestive issues and creates havoc in your life. The Paleo diet is a good step toward a healthy body because the real food will save you from lots of health problems.

This book is designed as a guide for you so that you can learn about Paleo diet, meal plans. Exercise programs and common mistakes. If you want to follow a Paleo diet, then this book will be a good start for you.

Part 2

The Paleo Diet – An Introduction

If you look at the way the world is progressing it seems to be a world of copy cats and reengineers trying to relive the past. The same thing comes into play when you talk about diets and diet programs. It seems that every week a new diet comes out on the market that says the diet that came out last week is full of garbage. The new diet is the one everyone needs to be on. You can now eat what the old diet said you can't eat. To change your life, just buy this book and sign up to this gym or buy this new piece of equipment that will end up sitting in the corner of your house keeping your shirts and pants from hitting the floor no doubt. The newspapers are full of food scare stories. Chocolate is the new smoking and the next week it's bacon which is the villain of the piece. It's confusing!

Well, if you are tired of it as much as I am it is time to do something about it. It is time to take a stand and look at yourself, your life and what you want to do and how you want to do it. You need to get back to basics.

In this book I am NOT going to tell you about the greatest new fad or snazziest piece of equipment that will make your life easier. In fact I am going to do just the opposite. What I am going to be talking about in this book is something that has been lost through the passage of time. I am going to talk about a diet that our ancestors have known about and have almost forgotten about for hundreds of years. I am going to talk to you about a diet that wasn't really a diet in the traditional sense i.e. where you lose weight or which was designed to help weight loss. It was a diet that people consumed as their natural daily food intake.

IN THE BEGINNING

In the beginning we didn't have grocery stores or corner market. We didn't keep our food locked away in nice ice cold boxes that kept everything fresh. We didn't have prepackaged boxes with labels on them telling us our nutritional benefits. No, what we had were spears, rocks and our bare hands. We didn't have doctors telling us what to eat and what not to eat. What we had was our brains and our instinct. We ate for survival not for comfort or convince.

And you know what, we survived and we thrived. We grew into a mighty society where we have the advancements that we have today. We have the modern medicines that cure the sick and fix the injured. We have what we need to survive since we learned what it took to survive all those many years ago. Now in our modern age we need to step back and take a look at our past. We need to turn off the technology that makes our lives so comfortable and safe. We need to look at the teachings of our ancestors and move our way back to eating the way they did.

WHY

Why? Well it is simple. Back then our ancestors didn't have heart disease, hypertension, stress, cancer or any number of other diseases that you care to mention. Go back to your history books. Read about how life was back in the olden days. True, it was hard and people died of diseases all the time. But you need to look at those diseases. They were colds, influenza, dysentery, malaria, cuts and many others that were caused by poor living conditions not by their diet.

Now fast forward to the year 2000. What are we all dying of today? Cancer, heart disease, liver disease, diabetes and a slew of other diseases that didn't exist back then. Why is that? Well I am not a scientist and I am not a doctor, I am a health conscious Virgo who has been researching diets and food since I was 16 in order to resolve my asthma, allergies and the health problems of my loved ones. I think I have an advantage in not being a doctor as I have an untainted perspective and an open mind. A lot of doctors I know think diet has as much to do with your health as the music you listen to. Do you know that in their 7 years of training doctors only spend 6 weeks studying diet and food? I believe food is fundamental to our health and well-being.

I strongly believe that the additives and preservatives that are put into our foods along with modern mass production of food is contributing to ill health in the long and short term. Just think about it for a moment. If you went back in time and gave a caveman a Snickers do you not think he would roll over and die? I do. Why, because their bodies were not accustomed to all of those additives and preservatives. It is those additives and preservatives that are acting within our systems causing us not to be as healthy or fit as our ancestors.

The media often make out that health is a lottery and that those who are "struck down" - as they call it - with ill health are in some way victims of the this cruel, indiscriminate lottery game. I see it differently, you would never put an inferior petrol into your Porsche and expect it to run like a dream. You would not put a bar of soap into your dishwasher or moisturiser instead of fabric softener into your washing machine and expect good results and yet we abuse our body daily with high fat, high salt, high sugar processed meals which invite long terms health problems.

We can all dramatically improve our odds of good health by what we eat each day and the **Paleo Diet** is a fantastic way to start for all the reasons which will be outlined in the coming chapters.

So what are we to do?

Well, the truth is that we will not change overnight and if human history has anything to say about it we probably won't change until it is almost too late. But it is not your responsibility to worry about everyone else on the planet. It is your job to worry about you and your choices. This is why I decided to write this book and probably why you have decided to read it.

In this book I am going to introduce you to the Paleo Diet. The Paleo Diet or the caveman diet is what was eaten back in the days of the cave people. You know the dudes on the Gieco commercials. Well, anyway, I am going to walk you through their diet and why it is so beneficial for you to try it and see how you feel.

Now there will be no exercise equipment that you will need to buy and you don't have to go live in a cave to take full advantage of this diet but you will need to change your mindset and way of eating. Now, this is going to be a little hard for some, maybe even most of you to start off with and since we are so used to getting that pizza delivered to our houses with all of those great toppings. The only thing that I can tell you is that once you decide to take on this great diet you will start to feel better, act better and live longer and happier lives.

So if you are ready to take on this new adventure with me, I am ready to tell you everything that I know and probably a few things that I had to learn along the way. If you are ready to learn what our ancestors knew and thrived on then let's jump right into the Paleo Diet.

Let's GET STARTED, GET MOTIVATED AND FEEL GREAT!

The Paleo Diet - Covering The Basics

WHAT IS THE PALEO DIET?

Well this is the million dollar question isn't it? This is the main reason most of you purchased this book right? Well here it is in all of its glory. The Paleo Diet is the natural diet. The diet that our caveman ancestors ate all those many years ago.

Let's go back in time for a moment shall we. Just think back to when men and women lived in caves and small huts. They didn't have Wal-Mart's and Supermarkets to go to and get their foods. They couldn't go out and buy some microwave popcorn or order a pizza and have it delivered. No, our ancestors had to eat what was off the land. They didn't have the luxury of having the foods that we eat today.

And that is the problem isn't it - all the processed foods, all the fast foods, all the preservatives that we now have and use to make our lives more convenient. The problem is, that it isn't natural.

When you think of Paleo think of Paleolithic or the time of the cave man and dinosaurs. This is where we get the word Paleo from. The Paleolithic era was the time in human history where man had to survive off the land. They ate plants, small animals, fish and other natural things. They didn't have preserved meats or cans of soda and beer.

So that is what Paleo is. It is the natural way of eating.

WHY IS THE PALEO DIET A GOOD DIET?

Okay, so I guess you were wondering why, with all the pizza, hamburgers and hotdogs just a phone call away, why in the world would you want to go back to eating nuts and berries? Well there are many reasons.

First off, you are not going to be eating nuts and berries in caves. Second of all research into the bones found from our ancient ancestor's show that they had greater height, lifespans were longer and they appeared not to have suffered from the diseases and ailments of their grain eating decedents.

Well that sounds pretty good. Live longer and not have to worry about getting cancer or some other form of dread disease. So what do I eat on this magic diet?

WHAT TO EAT?

Okay, so the cavemen didn't have microwave popcorn, coffee, beer, crisps and all of those other great tasting foods in my cupboard. So does that mean I have to throw them out? I know you said I didn't have to eat nuts and berries, but I have to have my coffee in the morning and my husband has to have his beer? What are we going to do?

Okay, relax. I hear and feel you. I like my beer after a long day at work as well. Now the Paleo Diet is strict on some guidelines but it isn't so strict that if you want a cup of coffee or a beer or cupcake occasionally you cannot have it.

When you think of the Paleo Diet you need to think of it as a guideline not a Bible. You just need to learn guidelines and new certain habits.

Okay so what can I eat?

Organic meat

Fish and seafood

Eggs

Fresh fruit and vegetables

Seeds and nuts

Oils i.e. extra virgin olive oil, walnut oil, avocado, coconut, flaxseed and macadamia oil

What are the no-no's of Paleo?

Cereal Grains – Wheat, rice, millet, maize, oats, rye, quinoa, buckwheat, barley, sorghum, millet, semolina and fonio.

Legumes – Beans, lentils, peas, peanuts, alfalfa, soy beans.

Dairy

Sugar

Potatoes

Processed Foods

Salt

Refined Vegetable Oils.

What else to avoid?

Many condiments and seasonings contain gluten. One must eliminate all the following unless they specifically say that they are gluten free:

Worcester Sauce

MSG – MonoSodiumGlutomate

Malt products

Bouillon

Modified food starch

Barley malt

Soy Sauce

Salad Dressings or gravies thickened with wheat or gluten based products

What about alcohol?

Avoid:

Beer

Ale

Light beer

Check carefully your tolerance to alcoholic drinks distilled from gluten grains i.e. gin, whisky (scotch) and some vodka.

Anything else?

No processed meats

No sausages, hot dogs, cold meats, pepperoni, salami, polony, pate, hams, liverwurst, frankfurters and prosciutto. All these have cancer causing chemicals added and all are high in gluten due to the grains used in their manufacture.

"Oh heck, what will I eat?"

I know that many of you may already be scratching your heads as you contemplate a life without sandwiches, milkshakes, toast and morning cereals, but I am going to go through the list and explain why showing wheat, milk, sugar and salt the red card is the best thing you can do for your future.

Remember, try this diet for 30 days and you will be amazed at how your health and vitality improves and how many of your health issues resolve. You will look back on what once were staples and ask yourself how you ever ate them.

Through the rest of the book we will be exploring more about the Paleo Diet. We will give you some great recipes that you can try for yourself as well as give you resources that you can use to further your education.

The Paleo Diet is not necessary a diet to help you lose weight, even though most people do lose weight on Paleo. That is a huge misconception when it comes to the word diet. What the Paleo Diet is, is more of a lifestyle choice. Similar to vegetarians or vegans or whatever other group you want to mention. These people have chosen to step outside the confines of modern eating practices and turn towards a more natural way of eating. So if you are ready to go Paleo let's jump right in with both feet.

What Can Paleo Do For Me?

It is ideal for gluten intolerant people

It is ideal for dairy intolerant people

Reduces risk of heart disease, type II diabetes and many of the chronic dread diseases affecting those in the West.

Weight Loss

Improve or eliminate acne

Improve or eliminate psoriasis and eczema

Better fitness and energy level

Slows autoimmune illnesses

Better sleep

Improved libido

Better skin tone

Less problems with digestion i.e. heartburn, IBS

A healthier lifestyle.

Studies

The Department of Medicine within the University of California San Francisco School of Medicine, set up an outpatient study with nine volunteers.

The study involved comparing the health of those on a Paleo style diet rich in lean meat, vegetables, fruits and nuts with those on a diet rich in grains, dairy and legumes.

The results were remarkable.

The Paleo group experienced: lower blood pressure; improved arterial function, more balanced cholesterol levels and insulin improvements.

The Paleo diet works with your body's genetics to help you stay fit, healthy and full of energy.

Research in biochemistry, biology, dermatology, ophthalmology and many more clinical disciplines indicate that the 21st century diet rich in processed food, sugar and bad fats is the root of all degenerative diseases i.e. cancer, diabetes, heart disease, Parkinson's, Alzheimer's and also inextricably linked to IBS, infertility, ADD, autism and depression.

Can It Work For Diabetes?

In a test with a group of participates eating Paleo and another eating the Mediterranean style diet the Paleo group reversed the signs and signals of insulin resistant Type 2 diabetes, while the Mediterranean Diet showed very little if any improvement.

One can read the research here: http://www.staffanlindeberg.com/DiabetesStudy.html

Lean meat proteins support muscles, bones and the immune function and help keep you full and satisfied between meals.

While giving up dairy and wheat may seem like giving up all your staples and the foods you have grown up to believe are good for you, I believe that the Western Diet has become over dependent on wheat and milk to the degree that they now form a much larger percentage of our daily intake than they should and often at the expense of fruit and vegetables. Wheat based products are also highly processed and the more processed food is, the more acidic it becomes.

On a day to day basis our eating revolves around wheat and diary. In the morning it's cereals with milk or butter on toast. Lunch is cheese sandwiches. Yogurt as a snack. Dinner may be pasta with a creamy, cheesy sauce. The Paleo diet offers a very healthy alternative to this pattern of wheat and dairy intake which can made a huge difference to your health and weight.

They also say that one man's meat is another man's poison. Everyone is unique and a new diet may affect one person in a different way to another as our metabolisms are all very different; there is no doubt however that including more fruit and vegetables into your diet and reducing the amount of processed foods is never a bad thing.

Eating Paleo works for many people who are looking to lose weight and increase their overall sense of well-being. It does make sense from an evolutionary point of view in terms of how our digestion was designed.

Paleo Is Rich In Omega-3

Omega rich fats from nuts, seeds, avocados, olive oil, fish oil and organic grass fed meat greatly support a healthy immune system.

Scientific research has shown that diets rich in Omega-3 fats and other monounsaturated fats dramatically reduce the instances of obesity, cancer, heart and cognitive disease.

Flaxseed oil, walnuts, Brussels sprouts, kale, spinach and salad greens all contain omega 3.

The long chain fats of Omega 3 are channelled to form cell wall membranes which fight systemic inflammation and boost the body's immune responses. The modern Western diet which tends to be so overloaded with processed food is deficient in Omega 3 and often we get too much Omega 6 instead leading to an imbalance that promotes disease.

A Research Team from the University of Manchester in a paper published in the American Journal of Clinical Nutrition demonstrated that taking Omega 3 fish oils could help protect against skin cancer. Trials are under way.

A team of Chinese researchers published their findings on Omega 3 and breast cancer risk reduction in the British Medical Journal (BMJ). They assert that a high intake of the Omega 3 fats found in fish are associated with a 14% reduction in the risk of breast cancer later in life. In the study they reviewed and analysed a collection of 26 studies done in the US, EU and Asia involving over 800,000 participants and 20,000 cases of breast cancer.

Omega 3 supports heart, brain, mood, joint, skin, immune and vision health. The eyes and brain contain a significant level of DHA, which is the mature form of Omega 3. DHA improves nerve cell growth and communication.

Omega 3 supplementation benefits depression, anxiety, stress, ADHD, bi-polar and many more of the common mental problems we hear more and more about and which did not seem to affect our ancestors as dramatically.

Omega 3 deficiency is a risk factor in major psychiatric and personality disorders and also suicide and homicide.

Arthritis is relieved by Omega 3.

Organic meat is lower in saturated fat

Saturated fat has been the health and well-being bogeyman for many years. Why has the saturated fat content of our diets increased over the generations?

The amount and type of fat found within grain fed as opposed to grass fed livestock or wild animals is striking. Wild meat is very lean with less trace of saturated fat, while being rich in Omega-3 fats like EPA and DHA. Professor Cordain in his paper Saturated Fat and consumption in Ancestral Die, reaches the conclusion that free range meat is far healthier than conventional meat in terms of the ratio of saturated to healthy fats present.

Concerns about wheat and other grains have been growing over the past two decades and I feel that since many of the grains we consume will soon be genetically modified, there is more reason than ever to purge one's diet of these grains.

Celiac disease which is a chronic gut infection which destroys the intestinal villi and thereby the body's ability to absorb nutrients is on the rise – quite a dramatic rise actually.

Gluten toxicity which brings on Celiac disease and other autoimmune reactions i.e. allergies, occurs mostly due to peptides within gluten which damage the intestinal tract.

If untreated Celiac disease leads to malnutrition and other severe concerns i.e. chronic fatigue and mental disorders.

Reactions to gluten can occur within hours or days later. Gluten intolerance can also lead to rheumatoid arthritis or Crohn's disease as well as a multitude of the ailments i.e. irritable bowel syndrome, headaches, eczema or psoriasis. Sprue is a form of debilitating arthritis usually accompanied by a host of digestive symptoms and is caused by eating gluten.

If you are saying to yourself, "My grandparents and their grandparents ate wheat and there was nothing wrong with their health," do bear in mind that wheat contained only 5% gluten 50 years ago and now it contains 50% gluten due to the fact it has be hybrid to resist fungus and grow quicker to feed a population which has exploded.

The bottom line in any industry is satisfying demand and covering costs, thus production efficiency and volume often override the health consequences. Bread, cakes, rolls, muffins etc. are mass produced as fast as possible to keep the shelves of supermarkets stocked and a constant stream of sweet treats going to cafes and coffee shops. These hastily produced wheat products are filled with additives and inferior ingredients and short cuts in their production add to their toxicity.

High speed methods of baking which have evolved over time involve adding toxic additives and mixing the dough violently so that loaves can be baked, cooled, packaged and sent out within hours. Certainly not how it was done back in the 'old days' of our grandparents.

It was when I started suffering severe eczema that I realised that anything 'baked' from a supermarket or coffee shop was the cause; I became very curious in what indeed I was eating.

Agriculture has had to keep up with the growing demand for wheat and so the hybrid process was sped up to cater for the baking industry's requirement for pliable proteins, leading to wheat containing 10 times the gluten it once did.

Sugar – The Devil You Know

Do you remember the advertising campaign of the 80's, "Sugar gives you go!"

Well it should rather have been, "Sugar has to go!"

Eating sugar is a dietary no-no, as not only is it bad for your teeth and weight gain, it could be significantly adding to your chance of developing cancer.

Over the past 50 years the increase in sugar consumption has been exponential, partly due to the use of high fructose corn syrup (HFCS) in processed food and the increased sucrose content in our day food and beverages.

Sucrose and HFCS hide everywhere from sauces to savoury foods and so it is vital to read the label. As the natural food fibre is removed from the sugar, it is fast tracked into our bloodstream where it makes us feel good by giving us a boost of energy. Sugar masks unpleasant flavours, adds to shelf life and is addictive so we eat far more than we need to.

It isn't just calories, it's poison.

Sugar contributes far more to obesity than dietary fat.

Obesity, diabetes, cancer and coronary disease and other health issues have become epidemic since the 50's and it seems the link to our intake of sugar could not be more clear.

Research published in the journal Nature Medicine has confirmed that processed sugar is one of the key drivers behind the growth and spread of cancer tumours, to the extent that cancer screening could rely on scanning the body for sugar accumulation in the future. "Tumours consume much more glucose than normal, healthy tissues in order to fuel their growth," according to a recent University College London (UCL) announcement. Sugar can trigger and promote cancer at even low levels. Sugar is the primary and the preferred fuel for cancer cells.

Many malignant tumours respond directly to the insulin that is produced when we consume sugar. The UCL study is not a lone voice in establishing a connection between cancer and sugar: Dr. Robert H. Lustig, M.D., a Professor of Paediatrics in the Division of Endocrinology at the University of California, San Francisco (UCSF), confirms that the majority of chronic illnesses plaguing humankind right now are caused by sugar consumption.

Hormones which are produced in the body in response to sugar intake actually feed the cancer cells. Whenever you down a fizzy drink or a bar of chocolate, chemicals are produced which encourage cancer cells to grow in size and spread.

Regular moderate consumption of sugary foods and beverages along with a diet containing refined carbohydrates, can lead to the onset of many chronic diseases. Dementia and diabetes have been linked to dietary sugar and now there is evidence that excess sugar over the decades can dramatically increase the risk of heart failure.

Other problems with sugar

Although natural unprocessed sugar has some nutrients, the processing of sugar for daily use involves the inclusion of many harmful chemicals. Processed sugar and fructose have absolutely no mineral content and they actually leech minerals off our body and from our teeth. They inhibit the absorption of minerals especially magnesium which is vital for over 300 metabolic processes.

The Candida yeast infection which exists in the gut of everyone, can begin to grow like a weed when fuelled by food containing sugar and yeast. It begins to overwhelm the friendly bacteria in the gut and it eventually spreads throughout the body producing health problems i.e. eczema, allergies, asthma, IBS, chronic fatigue and many more. Cancer will thrive in a Candida environment.

Sugar is addictive. It creates an immediate kick by stimulating the central nervous system neurotransmitters dopamine and serotonin, you are thus encouraged to eat more and more of it even if you are no longer hungry.

None of us can avoid sugar totally and to have a treat now and again is fine; I have tried here to give you enough good reasons to kick sugar out of your daily routine and keep it for a treat only.

Dairy, Dairy Quite Contrary.

Cow's milk was meant for calves not humans.

Did you ever think about the fact that humans are the only mammals which drink another specie's milk?

The milk one buys at the dupermarket is packed with hormones and provides far less calcium and vitamins than other food stuffs. Did you spot the typo – dupermarket? I think supermarkets should be called dupermakets as we are being duped into buying products which purport to be good for us when they are not.

Flavoured milks, yogurts and dairy products are also loaded with sugar.

Milk contains about 60 hormones, a plethora of allergens, fat, cholesterol and scientists have theorised that there is a link between milk and the switching on and off of cancer genes.

"Thatcher Thatcher the milk snatcher."

In the 70's when Margaret Thatcher was education minister she stopped the free milk given to all school children. This is still talked about today as a 'bad thing' and it does demonstrate how ingrained it is in our culture that milk is good for you. There are many other foods which contain more calcium and a superior nutritional value than milk i.e. green leafy vegetables, wild salmon, almond and coconut milk

Plant based sources of calcium and vitamin D are absorbed far more efficiently than animal based sources, and are much healthier

Cheeses and yogurts are highly processed and high in either sodium, sugar or aspartame.

Milk may worsen asthma in children due to either an undiagnosed milk allergy or by stimulating excess mucous production in the lungs.

For anyone with a lung condition, mucous forming dairy products are best avoided

"In all respiratory conditions, mucous-forming dairy foods, such as milk and cheese, can exacerbate clogging of the lungs and should be avoided," writes Professor Gary Null in his Complete Encyclopaedia of Natural Healing.

As Dr. Robert M. Giller writes in Natural Prescriptions, eliminating dairy from the diets of many adult and child asthma sufferers helps. "not because dairy products stimulate mucus production but because they're very common causes of allergy, upper-respiratory allergies and asthma (which may be an allergy in itself)."

Teenage and adult acne improves within weeks of one giving up milk and dairy. Androgens in cow's milk stimulate the sebaceous glands, which are the glands that cause the acne.

Were you born in the 50's, 60's or 70's? Ask your Mom about Dr. Spock.

Dr. Spock was a household name back in the day and his book on childcare sold 75 million copies, second only to the Bible in terms of sales. Dr. Spock said that no human, no child and no adult needed cow's milk.

What are the five biggest health problems facing Americans? Heart disease, osteoporosis, cancer, diabetes and asthma. If we consider nations where dairy consumption is high we find a direct correlation. In the UK, France, Canada and the US cheese consumption has tripled in the last 30 years and there has also be a tripling of the occurrences of asthma and breast cancer.

The country with the highest breast cancer rate in the world is Denmark, followed by Norway, Holland and Sweden. These four countries also have the highest rates of heart disease. It is no coincidence that dairy consumption in these four countries are the highest in the world.

China, where milk was traditionally a small part of the diet, has had a very low breast cancer rate.

1000's of things cause cancer and the Daily Express and Daily Mail delight in headlines which reveal either what causes it or the latest miracle cure. There are mechanisms by which diseases like cancer occur. Many things may cause it, however one thing makes it grow and that is the insulin growth factor: the most powerful growth factor in your body. An in a remarkable scientific twist of fate that specific hormone in a human and a cow's body is identical. Out of 4700 species of mammal and billions of different proteins in nature, only one hormone in the entire animal kingdom is identical between two species: human and cow IGF-1. IGF-1 has been identified as a key factor in the growth and proliferation of breast, lung, prostrate and many other cancers.

But these hormones are destroyed by pasteurisation right? Milk is homogenised: meaning that the fat molecules are made from 10 to 100 times smaller. The fat molecules envelop and protect the hormones meaning that they can remain reactive in the human body for up to 30 minutes, during which time they can act as a turn on mechanism for cancer.

And remember it takes 10 pounds of milk to make one pound of hard cheese and 21 to make a pound of butter.

I hope you do not think that this is all one big scare story! Milk and dairy products are being **over** consumed by people in the Western world – again, an ice cream or a pizza now and again won't harm you, however a heavily dairy dependant diet is just not healthy.

The good news is that almond, hazelnut, rice and oat milks are now readily available as are a range of vegan cheeses. The problem is that these can contain sugar and since they are processed, there is the danger of additives – read the label and use with caution.

Would You Put Chip Pan Oil In Your Ferrari?

Of course not, so why are you using rancid unhealthy oils in your kitchen?

Switching away from bad oils is EASY!

Corn, canola (rapeseed oil) and soybean oil were never meant for human consumption. They were manufactured for industrial purposes i.e. lubrication or for the next generation of car fuel. They are cheaper to produce than healthy fats and oils and have many profitable by-products.

Although the small amounts of oil found in wholegrain corn and soybeans are healthy, as a mass produced product, the oil is required to have a longer shelf life. The fatty acids in grains turn rancid quickly and so to make them last, the phytochemicals and antioxidants which prevent them from being dangerous oils are removed. The oil is processed using bleach and hexane, thereafter it is deodorised. Colorants, flavourings and other chemicals are often added to mask the natural smell.

The health impact of these oils ranges from: disruption to the central nervous system, anaemia, loss of vision, respiratory illnesses, constipation and mental issues. In the longer term there is the increased risk of cancer, heart attack, stroke, digestive disorders and vitamin deficiency.

What's more, canola oil comes from crops which are increasingly genetically modified. Rapeseed is easy to grow successfully as it is so toxic even insects don't want it. GM rapeseed or canola oil has been linked to lung cancer and heart disease.

Soybean oil also has a dark side and has been linked to cancer, infertility and infantile leukaemia.

Long term use of corn oil can promote colon cancer. Japanese researchers discovered that corn oil use was associated with shorter lifespans and oesophageal cancer.

These dangerous oils lurk in the system and their effects are usually only long term in nature; this is why they are so dangerous. In the short term they are innocuous, but the cumulative effect over years can be dramatic.

Switching to cold pressed, extra virgin oils with medium chain fatty acids can reduce the risk of heart disease, cancer and many other ailments.

Legumes – Not What It Says On The Box.

You have all seen the benefit of 'whole-grain' extolled on the TV screens. Many of these so called whole grain cereals and products are loaded with sugar and few are in fact 100% whole grain. These grains may be doing you more harm than good. Grains, legumes and nuts are not pret-a-manger! The fibre from whole grains is tough and can actually increase digestive difficulties. They can contribute to IBS, Crohn's disease and inflammatory bowel disease as well as to constipation and many more disorders of the digestive tract.

A diet rich in whole grains, especially wheat can damage the digestive system leading to allergies, celiac disease, mental illness and an overgrowth of the Candida fungus as mentioned in the section on sugar. There is even evidence of a link between gluten and multiple sclerosis.

Another problem with legumes and some nuts and seeds is that they contain phytic acid, an anti-nutrient. Phytic acid contributes to mineral deficiencies, namely calcium, magnesium, iron and zinc deficiency. Tannin is another nasty found in legumes: tannins irritate the digestive tract. Enzyme inhibitors found in legumes and grain place stress on the pancreas.

Wheat and gluten hide in most processed foods including medicines and supplements, so one must read the labels carefully. Gluten intolerance often goes undiagnosed as symptoms are wide ranging. If you suffer indigestion, allergies, bloating, constipation or eczema, try going gluten free and you may just change your life.

"No netball until you drink your milk!"

So, there you have the low down on all those foods the media told you were your best friends and in some cases the foods your folks forced down you for your own good – they thought. I know that for some people it can be hard to accept that the food staples you were brought up with are at the root of your health issues, but it's time to rethink and reshape your thinking.

REVOLUTIONIZE YOUR LIFE AND YOUR HEALTH WITH PALEO.

History Of Paleo

As I stated earlier the Paleo diet is the diet that our ancestors ate back in the Stone Age. The main reason that they ate this diet is because they had not yet perfected or come up with agriculture. No one knows the origin of the Paleo diet or why it was eaten, but back in 1913 a man going by the name of Joseph Knowles conducted an amazing experiment that would change the way we thought of food and the way we eat.

Mr. Knowles experiment was to see what would happen if we went back to the way our caveman ancestors ate. So he took some minimal requirements such a tent, bedding and some basic comforts, I mean it was an experiment on eating habits not living habits after all, and lived off the land for a period of two months.

When Mr. Knowles came back and released his findings he stated that he had felt better than he had in his entire life. He stated that he had more energy, felt stronger and fit as well as had a more positive outlook on life. When asked by his peers what he believed was the cause of this amazing transformation Mr. Knowles stated that it was from his diet.

After his return Mr. Knowles stated that the sudden urbanization of America and American living has taken us away form a healthy way of living and that we needed to return to that lifestyle if we as a society were to prosper into a healthy future.

Now it wouldn't be until many years later that the official term "Paleo Diet" was coined. This honor has been given to a gentleman going by the name of Walter L. Voegtin. Mr. Voegtin coined this phrase in his book "The Stone Age Diet" which was published in 1975. In his book he argued that the human race was carnivorous in nature and that we needed to revert back to that lifestyle. He stated that if we wanted perfect health that we needed to go back to the diet our ancestors had. He went on to say that those in this time period were fit, trim and lived healthier and happier lives.

Mr. Voegtin also believed that since modern man received 99.99% of genic blueprint from our Stone Age ancestors, that we are naturally engineered to be on this diet and not the diet that we as a society are currently on.

Now like many other great innovations of the past, the words fell on deaf ears. Back in the 1970's people were more interested in peace and love and expanding their minds with other distractions other than healthy eating. But like everything else in life, times change and with books and articles being written in the 80's, 90's and today people are starting to look at the wisdom of the past as well as the ways things were done. One of those changes is the reexamination of the Paleo diet and what it can do for us as a society.

So What Is The Paleo Diet Anyway?

Now I bet you have been waiting for this section since you decided you wanted to take on the Paleo diet. The food is the most important part when it comes to a diet. People don't want to be eating nuts, berries, protein shakes with green chunks of whatever that stuff is floating around in there, without knowing why. They want to eat what they want to eat when they want to eat it. And I don't blame them one bit.

When it comes to food people want to eat what tastes good, makes them satisfied and is quick and easy. We don't want to eat stuff that is complicated or makes the neighbors put their houses up for sale from the stench coming from your kitchen because you decided to start eating "healthy".

So in this section we will talk to you more about the foods that are on the Paleo diet. We will tell you what is good and what is not good. Then from there you can decide on what you want to eat and what you don't.

I will highlight in bold everything you can eat for quick reference.

PROTEIN

Now we all love our protein. I know I do and so did my caveman brothers and sisters.

When it comes to protein on the Paleo diet here are the items that you will want to add to your diet.

Meat, offal or organ meat, poultry, fish, seafood and eggs. **These items are what you will want to have on a daily basis. From there you can add other items on an occasional basis. These foods include cured meats such as** bacon, sausage and ham. **Since curing meat adds salt and salt wasn't a real concern to those back in the Stone Age, it really isn't a part of their diet. Always buy organic when possible. When buying sausages check what percentage is actually meat and not gluten-rich filler. Smoked meats often have added ingredients which are highly allergic and so be careful.**

The proteins that you will never want to add to your diet are the following:

Legumes which are beans and lentils. Those back in this time did not have beans available to them on a regular basis so adding them to the Paleo diet is a no no.

Soy and tofu. Now personally I think that tofu is gross and so waving that goodbye was a slam-dunk. I like soy sauce for my rice as it is salty, but again, it is not part of the Paleo diet. Sorry...

Vegetable protein is another no-no on the list as well as peanuts and meats that are breaded or prepared with grains. You also don't want to add sugars to your foods or cook anything in vegetable or seed oils. If you stick to these guidelines you will be eating Paleo.

FATS

As Oprah once said, "What does fat do other than make everything taste better?"

Now who doesn't like fat? Fat is one of the reasons that I get up in the morning. Well, not really but it does taste good. In today's society we eat and or consume a lot of fats in our diets. Now some fats are good and some fats are bad. There is a raging debate on what good fat is and what bad fat is. There is a debate on Tran's fats, cholesterol levels, good cholesterol, bad cholesterol and the list goes on and on. Honestly I don't think the experts even know what a good fat is and what a bad fat is. I feel that it has gotten so commercial and so blurred that no one really knows anything anymore. This is another good reason why going back to the basics and starting all over with your diet is such a good thing. Aren't you glad you decided to learn about Paleo?

Anyway, here are the fats that you should be adding to your diet on a daily basis.

You want to start off with **lard, tallow and duck fat**. Yep, you heard me duck fat. From there you want to add **Ghee, coconut oil, palm oil and macadamia oil**. You can also add avocado and **avocado oils** to your diet and finally olives and **olive oil**.

Then on a limited basis you can add nut oils i.e. **walnut** to your foods. Since our cavemen friends didn't really make oils out of nuts we don't want to add them to our diets en masse.

And finally you want to **avoid** the following fats all together in your diet: vegetable and seed oils. These oils include but are not limited to soybean oil, canola oil, cottonseed oil, corn oil, sunflower oil, safflower oil (never come across of that one personally), grape seed oil and finally peanut oil. Also added to that list are shortening and margarines.

DRINKS

The next items we will talk about are what the Stone Age man drank. This is something that most of us never really thought about. Since we have such a wide variety of items that we can drink from juice, soda, beer or whatever else is out on the market today from the makers of Pepsi and Coke, it is hard to imagine what the caveman drank. Well here comes a shock ladies and gentlemen, if you are going to go on the caveman diet you will be limiting your drinking options. Sorry.

When it comes to the Paleo diet you are limited to drinking the following items. **Water (filtered or sparkling).** We have too much junk in our modern day water (in London the water has passed through about 6 kidneys before you drink it) so you will need to get bottled water or buy one of those filtering systems i.e. Brita. Tap water also contains hormones as a result of people taking the pill, whereby the hormones land up in drinking water.

From there you can **drink tea and bone broths**. I suggest **natural fruit juices with no added sugar**, but these must be watered down by 50% at least. The juices one buys at the store are highly concentrated. You would not eat 15 oranges or 10 peaches at once and so drinking a highly concentrated fruit juice is just as silly. This simply supplies the body with way too much fructose and yes...that is fattening and unhealthy.

But didn't you say I can have my coffee in the morning and my husband can have his beer in the evening when he gets home from a hard day's work? Yes I did. You can have coffee on an occasional basis and you can drink "beer" / "alcohol" as long as it is gluten free.

What you can't drink is alcohol that contains gluten, soft drinks (including Coke Zero and Pepsi Max), nor any other type of beverage that contains sugars or artificial sweeteners, colors or anything else "modern science" has added to our drinks. It is all natural people.

Green smoothies and juice you make yourself with a juicer is fine in moderation.

PLANT FOODS

Remember back in the beginning when I told you that you didn't have to eat nuts and berries on this Paleo diet. Well you're right. You don't have to. In fact some nuts and berries aren't even on the Paleo diet to start with. With that being said here are what is and what is not on the Paleo diet vegetable lists.

What should you be eating on a daily basis? You should eat **vegetables, tubers and fruits**. What you should add occasionally to your diet are nuts and nut butters. These include nuts such as **almonds, hazelnuts, walnuts, macadamia nuts, Brazil nuts, pistachios,** and a few others.

The items you need to stay away from are gluten containing grains which include wheat, barley, (beer) rye, as well as some oats. Some of the non-gluten items that you will want to stay away from are corn, oats, rice, quinoa, sorghum, buckwheat and amaranth.

Some of the main foods you want to stay away from **are bread, pasta, oatmeal, breakfast cereals, pizza, granola bars, tortillas, cakes (yep even chocolate cake), pizza, pasta, cookies and other baked goods (no ovens back then either).**

Well, I know I probably lost half of you on the alcohol part and probably another good hunk of you on the cake part but for the rest of you who have stuck it out this far I only have one more misc. section to tell you about and then you can decide if the Paleo diet is something that you can live on.

MISC.

In this section we will wrap up what can and can't be eaten on the Paleo diet. I hope that I haven't scared you all away with the last few sections but this section will be relatively harmless.

Items that you **should be adding** to your diet are **spices and herbs**. These items not only make your food taste better in many cases they offer a healing aspect to the body. You will want to **add vinegar as well as fermented vegetables**.

Other items that you will want to **add occasionally** to your diet are fermented dairy if you can handle dairy, I am not exactly sure how or why you would drink **fermented dairy** but in some cultures it is popular. **Dark chocolate** but it has to be at least 70% coco (and not added to a cake, sorry), **unprocessed sugar** which include **raw honey and maple syrup**.

Items that you can't eat are sugars which include white sugar, brown sugar, agave syrup, high fructose corn syrup or HFCS. You don't want to eat anything that has any form of chemical ingredients or artificial sweeteners.

When it comes to the Paleo diet it really just comes down to what the cavemen ate. If it is something that was eaten off the land before the advent of modern technology or agricultural advances then it could be considered to be Paleo. If it is food that does not have something artificial added to it and or wasn't engineered by man then it can be considered to be on the Paleo diet.

The Crucial Do's And Don'ts

So how are you enjoying Paleo so far? Is it everything you thought it would be? Are you excited about the benefits?

Are you eagerly awaiting the recipe section of this book so you can get started on your journey into eating Paleo? Well don't start getting all Paleo on me yet as there is a lot more I need to tell you about this diet. In this section I am going to be breaking down the dos and don'ts of Paleo.

Rules! Oh man, you already gave me a buzz kill on the coffee and cake what else are you going to throw at me? Don't worry it will be painless. There are only twelve do's and don'ts when it comes to Paleo. Just think of it as your twelve step program to living a better healthier life.

Ready, here we go.

#1 – EAT PLENTY OF MEAT

Okay, this one shouldn't be a problem for people especially if you love steak and chicken. When eating meat you will want to eat beef, lamb, poultry, pork, organic meat, fish, and seafood. Eat organic whenever possible. When getting these items you will want to stay away from the meats that are pumped with hormones and other chemicals which help increase size and other aspects of the animal. When getting your meat I suggest going to a meat market or a butcher. I started doing this and it not only saves me money during the month but the food tastes better.

#2 – EAT A LOT OF EGGS

Now I love eggs. I have at least three or four in the morning for breakfast. Now some people advocate removing the yolk from the eggs since they say it contains too much cholesterol. Well don't do that. You want to eat the egg yolks. The more yolks the better. Now, if you are worried about saturated fat don't. Also, if you are a vegetarian as well as trying to go Paleo you will want to eat eggs to help with muscle production and fat loss.

#3 – EAT A WIDE VARIETY OF VEGETABLES

The easiest way to shop is to follow this rule: "See a vegetable, buy it!"

If you are on the Paleo diet you will want to eat vegetables and a wide variety of vegetables at that. Cabbage is a hugely versatile and tasty vegetable.

You can slice or julienne any number of different veggies to make stir fries. Simply add sliced beef, chicken or fish to your stir fry for an amazing meal. I use any of these veggies in stir fries and different combinations give different flavors: zucchini, spring onions, charlotte onions, carrots, broccoli, cabbage, kale, shredded Brussels sprouts, green beans, red pepper, garlic, chives, coriander, pak choi, spinach, lemon grass, fresh basil and tomato.

When it comes to vegetables you will want to focus on cauliflower, carrots, bell peppers, tomatoes, cucumber, broccoli, Brussels sprouts, turnips, watercress, spinach, parsnips, kale, beets, yellow squash, pak choi, zucchini, and the list goes on and on. So when your mom told you all those years ago that you needed to eat your vegetables she was starting you on the path to Paleo. Thanks mom!

For loads of veggie rich soup and salad ideas that can be Paleo adapted try this book:

DELICIOUS and NUTRITIOUS RECIPES for the time and cash strapped
#4 – EAT HEALTHY FATS

Yes, there is good fat and bad fat. You want to focus on healthy fats. In case you forgot what some of those fats are from above here is a short reminder. Lard, tallow and duck fat Ghee, coconut oil, palm oil, macadamia oil, olive, avocado and walnut oil just to name a few. So when you are looking to add a little fat to your diet you need to refer to the ones listed.

#5 –CHOOSE QUALITY OVER PRICE.

When it comes to choosing meats you want to make sure that you choose quality meats. When you purchase a lower grade piece of meat you are actually purchasing all of the additives and preservatives that come along with modern culture. To eat Paleo you need to remove yourself from that manner of eating. When it comes to choosing your meat you want to go to places that specialize in meat. Yeah, going to Wal-Mart is easier but you are sacrificing quality over quantity. Consider going to a meat market or a butcher or a health food store. Yes you will be paying more but you get what you pay for not what you bargained for.

#6 – EAT MODERATE QUANTITIES OF FRUIT

You want to focus on berries. I know, I know, I said you didn't have to eat nuts and berries on this diet, just hear me out. When eating fruit you will want to focus on blueberries, blackberries and strawberries. Now one of the cool things about eating berries is that if you decide to eat blueberries you will be eating one of the top super foods that you possibly can. Why do you think there are blueberries in everything from pancakes to muffins? So add berries and other fruits to your diet.

#7 – STAY AWAY FROM STARCHY VEGETABLES

When you eat vegetables with starch the starch will convert to glucose which converts to fat. So if your goal on the diet is to lose weight you will want to stay away from foods with starch especially vegetables like squashes and potatoes.

#8 – STAY AWAY FROM GRAINS

Grains can be great (only when properly soaked and cooked) but the cavemen didn't eat them. Also, grains are a source of inflammation, so if you have aches and pains you need to stay away from these grains. Another reason why you will want to stay away from grains is that they contain carbs. Now no matter what diet book you read they will tell you to stay away from carbs. Over consumption of carbs will lead to glucose production which turns into fat which is not good. So stay away from grains.

#9 – AVOID SUGAR

If you read the package label on any form of food there is bound to be some sort of sugar in it. Now this is one reason why you want to stay away from preprocessed foods. When you read the ingredients on the side of the package you will see that there is 0g of sugar which is true but they hide the sugar in artificial sweeteners and in other coded words.

When you eat sugar it will convert into glucose which is not good. The glucose will turn into fat when not used by the body.

#10 – AVOID LEGUMES

"Beans, beans the magical fruit." Isn't that what they say? I like my beans just as much as the other guy, especially when you mix them with beef. But when it comes to the Paleo diet, it is a no no. If you do have to eat beans though you might want to limit them to green beans or sugar snap beans.

#11 – AVOID VEGETABLE AND SEED OILS

You want to avoid all seed oils and vegetable oils. These oils were not part of the caveman diet and should not be a part of your diet as well. I know that most people like to eat out and of course how can you have a social life if you don't eat out? But when you eat out you really can't control what they cook with, but you can always ask. When it comes to cooking at home though, you can easily swap your cooking oils to ones that fall within the Paleo scale.

#12 – AVOID DAIRY PRODUCTS

Now I know we have gone round and round with this in this book but here is the thing: caveman didn't have domesticated cows so getting milk wasn't really an option. Secondly we put a lot of chemicals and preservatives in our milk to allow it to keep longer. You want to stay away from low fat milk, skim milk, low fat yogurt and any other form of processed milk product.

Cream in your coffee once a week is actually fine! Good news at last!

Well I hope you are learning a lot about Paleo and the Paleo diet and beginning to see that there are loads of delicious things you can still eat. In the next section of the book we will give you some cool recipes that you can start with to get your taste buds adapted to the Paleo diet.

The Sensational Paleo Celebrities

Hollywood always seems to be ahead of the game when it comes to health foods. In 'The Business' you have to look great, stay thin and stay young and so if they are doing it out there on Sunset Boulevard, we should be sitting up and taking notice.

When you are in front of the camera on a daily basis and have a lot of people looking at you and talking about you, looking and feeling good is top priority. So, with that being said why are celebrities going on the Paleo diet?

Well it is simple. It is the diet that gets results. Now you don't have to take my word for it, you can do your research on the Internet and see for yourself. In this section of the book I am going to talk about ten celebrities that are on the Paleo diet and what they think about it.

JAKE OSBOURNE

MEGAN FOX

JESSICA BIEL

MILEY CYRUS

MATHEW McCaughey

EVA LA RUE

URSULA GROBLERR

BECCA BORAWSKI

NOVAK DJOKOVIC

ANDREW FLINTOFF

So if you love them, if you hate them or even if you love to hate them you have to take notice when someone on the famous side of the fence takes on a diet. So let's see what they have to say.

JAKE OSBOURNE

Jake Osborne is the son of famous rock star Ozzie Osborne. At the age of 26 Jake was diagnosed with MS. MS is a degenerative disease that over 400,000 people suffer from in America alone.

Not being one that follows the rules Jake decided to forego modern medicine and decided to look at the past and see what was available to those in the history who may have suffered from this disease. Through his research he came across the Paleo diet.

With his positive attitude Jake says, "Conquer and Overcome!"

Jake contributes his wellbeing to his mentor Dr. Terry Wahls. Dr. Wahls defeated the disease by treating it with food not medicine. The secret of good health is in what we eat and not what modern medicine says will cure us.

So if you are someone suffering from MS or some other disease you may want to take Jake's motto of "Conquer and Overcome" to heart and start down the path of healthy eating and see how it can help you with the medical issues you may suffer from.

MEGAN FOX

Now unless you really are a caveman and have been living under a rock for the past few years you must have heard of Megan Fox. Megan is the mega star in the Transformer movies. And if you have ever watched one of those movies you will know how sexy Megan looks. Well, when you are the star of a multi-million dollar movie you have to look good. I know, you go for the robots but you stay for the fox.

A Native American Megan knows how it is to live off the land. Megan knows that we all come from the earth and return to the earth and need it to sustain ourselves while we are here. This is one of the main reasons she is on the Paleo diet.

One of Megan's favorite foods is almonds. She eats them on an almost daily basis as a snack. Wife, mother, actress and Paleo diet supporter Megan Fox endorses the Paleo diet and thinks others should as well.

JESSICA BIEL

Even though she is a very busy person, Jessica Biel loves to cook homemade foods. The homemade foods that she loves to eat can be found on the Paleo diet. Jessica is quoted as saying, "I do a lot of cooking at home using fresh fish and lean meats like chicken as well as complimenting them with garden fresh vegetables."

Jessica just likes to eat healthy and doesn't believe in the word "DIET". Jessica believes that the Paleo diet is a way of living healthily and doesn't really help you lose weight but in fact just helps keep you trim and fit. "Everyone needs to lose a little water weight and keep those few extra pounds away so staying on the Paleo diet does that for me." – Author requoted and reworded.

If you are someone who wants to look as good as Jessica Biel as well as live the same healthy lifestyle, take a closer looks at the Paleo diet and Paleo lifestyle.

MILEY CYRUS

Miley Cyrus has been accused of having an eating disorder. The singer / actress seemed to have lost a lot of weight which resulted in the accusations. When pinned down Miley stated that she did not have an eating disorder but she had decided to change her eating lifestyle to the Paleo lifestyle.

When asked why she went Paleo, she stated that she went towards Paleo as she wanted to eliminate gluten from her diet. She also stated the changes to your mental health and body such as skin would be amazing and you wouldn't want to go back.

Finally she was quoted to saying, "It is not about weight it is about health"

So if you are a fan of Miley Cyrus or not, you should be a fan of her realizations when it comes to health and wellbeing. Why not try what she suggests? Go gluten free for one week and see how you feel. If you start to feel a little better go another week without eating gluten.

We all need to start to take better care of ourselves and if the ones we look up to and the ones our kids look up to are making a change towards Paleo then what is the harm in trying it yourself. There could be a lot worse things that we could be taking away from celebrities actions.

MATHEW MCCAUGHEY

Mathew is a big supporter of the Paleo diet. He believes in it so much that he has done everything he can to eliminate sugars and processed grains from his diet. He believes in fasting as well as doing everything he can to stay in shape.

Mathew stated that he is in the profession where his body is his tool and he wants to make sure that his body is in the best shape that it can be. "If I were not in shape then I would not be able to do what I needed to do."

But if you think that Mathew's house is one under military rule when it comes to not eating other than the Paleo way, you would be wrong. Mathew has been quoted as saying that he allows himself ten percent of his eating time to pigging out with his kids.

So if you are someone looking to take part in the Paleo lifestyle you can see that others do let their hair down every once and awhile. You do need to treat yourself to what the other half eat every now and again.

So be strict to a point but don't sacrifice enjoyment for health and health for enjoyment. Find a common ground like Mathew did.

EVA LA RUE

Television star on the hit television program CSI Miami has taken the principles of the Paleo diet and has run with them. Eva states that she has a hectic schedule that starts early in the morning and doesn't stop until late at night. Trying to juggle motherhood and a career, Eva can't afford to feel sluggish or start looking worn out and tired.

This is why she adopted the Paleo lifestyle. Calling it the "Paleo Solution" she embraces every aspect to its fullest.

URSULA GROBLER

"When I am close to a competition, I am super strict Paleo." - Ursula Grobler

Ursula is the current world record holder, as of 2014, in the indoor ergometer and the world's best lightweight rower. "It helps me keep the weight I need to compete as well as supporting good eating habits."

When a world record holder and athlete supports Paleo it is something. When you typically see athletes they are pounding down the carbs. Well this isn't the case with Ursula. She believes, and it shows, that cutting the carbs, sugars and additives out of her life, helps her look better, feel better and perform better than those who are on not on the Paleo diet.

So if you are striving to be a world record holder one day you may want to follow Ursula's example and move towards a Paleo diet.

BECCA BORAWSKI

"I only do it five to six days a week" – This is what Becca says when it comes to the Paleo diet. Being the program director of GetFit in LA, Becca needs to look her best and feel her best for her clients. If she doesn't look like she is happy and healthy her clients will take notice.

She is also quoted to have said that she has lower body fat, higher energy levels and better performance. All of these great factors she attributes to the transition to the Paleo lifestyle.

The Paleo diet is something that everyone should take a look at, at some point in their lives. We are so used to the common everyday diets that we are afraid to look for something that may be better. She also states that since the diet is rather restrictive that she only does it six days a week.

NOVAK DJOKOVIC

You do not have to be a tennis fan to have heard of Novak Djokovic, the tennis player with extraordinary stamina, strength, flexibility and fitness. He is the best athlete in world tennis.

In what he described as a life changing moment, Novak discovered that he was sensitive to gluten and diary – not great when your parents own a pizzeria as his do. Novak has not revealed that he is on Paleo as such, as that may be giving away too much info to his competitors; however after giving up gluten he said he felt lighter, slept better and was more energetic than he had ever been. When given a bagel to eat after one week gluten free, he said he immediately felt sluggish and dizzy as if he had a hangover.

Since swapping to a gluten and dairy free diet, Novak says he has felt stronger, lighter, more alert, mentally sharper and fresher.

Novak has tried many things from fitness regimes to meditation and yoga to address his problems with mid-match breakdown, which some had actually put down to asthma. All of these had some success, but nothing like the change in diet.

He now looks back to the point he gave up dairy, gluten and sugar as the turning point for him.

Novak's diet consists of vegetables, white meat, fish, nuts, seeds and healthy oils. He buys organic and cooks for himself whenever possible. Novak still eats legumes which are not really part of Paleo as you know, but I thought it was well worth including his experiences here.

ANDREW FLINTOFF

Professional boxer and retired cricket player Andrew Flintoff gave up that lifestyle of fighting and drinking alcohol a year ago for a cleaner lifestyle the Paleo way. "I am on the caveman diet!" he shouted to his friends and family. I have lost an amazing thirty (30) pounds so far on this diet and I am planning to lose an additional fifteen (15) pounds before I even consider going off this diet.

Andrew feels that he has never felt better or had a better outlook on life since he started eating the Paleo diet. "I wish I had known and adopted this diet years ago, I may have more championships under my belt."

FINAL CELEBRITY STATEMENT

In this past section I have told you about ten celebrities who have gone on the Paleo route and have stuck with it. Through their statements and lifestyle change they have endorsed the benefits and they will continue down the Paleo path for years to come.

Like I stated before, the Paleo diet is a lifestyle choice. We may make fun of celebrities for the way that they do things or make fun of them for the roles that they chose to play in movies, but when it comes to health and wellbeing actors and actresses use their bodies as their tools to make a living.

Just think about it for a moment. If you needed to look your best day in and day out with cameras on you at all times and tabloids and media questioning your every move, wouldn't you want to have something that supported you at all times?

I know I would. This is why the celebrities that I mentioned in this chapter have embraced the Paleo lifestyle. Now if they tried it and liked it why wouldn't you try it?

7 Days Of Paleo Eating – Breakfast, Lunch, Dinner And Snack Recipes

Okay, now we get into the food. I know what you have been thinking, everyone is raving about the Paleo diet but no one has told me exactly what they are eating. Now, when I go to the store I see meals for hundreds upon hundreds of weight loss plans and diet programs but I don't see anything that refers to the Paleo diet.

Now, if the Paleo diet was so good why don't they have a little box in the freezer section with a caveman on it telling me to buy their product? I mean I see a caveman on a cereal box and I see a caveman on television commercials but I don't ever hear any of them say the word Paleo. I do think I heard something close to that on a commercial with a lizard or something but I am pretty sure they weren't endorsing a food product.

Maybe after reading this chapter you can take my frozen Paleo food idea and try to market it, but in the mean time I have a seven day meal plan that you can follow in order to get started on the Paleo diet.

In the seven day meal plan I walk you through your entire day. I give you seven days' worth of food ideas that you can try. I start you off on Monday with breakfast, lunch, dinner, snack and dessert. Now of course you don't have to go day by day in order. You can jump around and mix and match different meal ideas. You can take a snack from day three and transpose it with day five. You can take the dinner idea on day seven and move it up to day one if you want. The choice is really up to you.

I hope that you enjoy my choices and that you don't feel like a caveman after eating these meals. If you find the Paleo diet does the business for you, you can find hundreds of recipes and meal choices online. Just Google "Paleo recipes" or "Paleo meal plans" for more ideas.

Enjoy.

DAY 1- MONDAY

BREAKFAST

LUNCH

DINNER

SNACK

DESSERT

DAY 2- TUESDAY

BREAKFAST

LUNCH

DINNER

SNACK

DESSERT

DAY 3- WEDNSDAY

BREAKFAST

LUNCH

DINNER

SNACK

DESSERT

DAY 4- THURSDAY

BREAKFAST

LUNCH

DINNER

SNACK

DESSERT

DAY 5- FRIDAY

BREAKFAST

LUNCH

DINNER

SNACK

DESSERT

DAY 6- SATURDAY

BREAKFAST

LUNCH

DINNER

SNACK

DESSERT

DAY 7- SUNDAY

BREAKFAST

LUNCH

DINNER

SNACK

DESSERT

Monday

Breakfast

Carrot Muffins

Servings 8

2 tsp. baking soda

Cinnamon

3 eggs

Apple cider vinegar

¾ c. walnuts

2 c. almond flour

Salt

1 c. dates, pitted

3 bananas

¼ c. coconut oil

1 ½ c. carrots grated

To start this recipe turn on the oven so it can heat up to 350 degrees (170C). Next, you take out a bowl and sift in the salt, flour, cinnamon, and baking soda. Set this bowl aside while you continue.

Taking out a blender: combine the vinegar, bananas, oil, eggs, and dates and then add this mixture to the dry ingredients and mix. Fold the carrots, dates and the nuts into the mixture and then spoon it all into your muffin tins.

After the tins are full, you can place them in the oven and allow the muffins to bake for 25 minutes. When the muffins are done cooking, you can take them from the oven and allow them some time to cool and then enjoy. Sprinkle with walnut pieces.

Nutritional Facts:

Calories 210

Fat 12g

Carbs 23g

Protein 3g

Lunch

Seafood Mint Salad

Servings 4

1 ½ c. shrimp

3 c. arugula/rocket

1 c. cubed mango

½ c. mint

1 c. cubed cantaloupe/sweet melon

3 Tbsp. lemon juice

1 tsp. nutmeg

1 tsp. cinnamon

Take out a salad bowl and combine together the lemon juice, nutmeg, cinnamon, mint, cantaloupe, mango, and shrimp, making sure to mix them together really well.

Serve on the rocket or arugula leaves.

Nutritional Facts

Calories 167

Fat 13g

Carbs 1g

Protein 23g

Dinner

Louisiana Fish

Servings 2

2 Tbsp. coconut oil

2 fish fillets

Juice from 1 lemon

Lemon pepper

Cayenne pepper

Garlic powder

Salt

Pepper

Preheat up the oven to about 350F (170C) degrees. While that is heating up you can heat up the lemon juice and the coconut oil gently in a corning ware dish or skillet. Place the fillets into the pan, making sure they are right next together so there is not much room leftover.

Take all of the spices and mix them together before sprinkling this seasoning on top of the fillets.

Bake the fillets for about 25 minutes before taking them out of the oven and giving them some time to cool down. Season the fillets with some pepper and salt if you wish before serving.

Serve with steamed broccoli and carrots or with a side salad of cucumber, cherry tomato, olives and lettuce.

Nutritional Facts

Calories 210

Fat 8g

Carbs 2g

Protein 25g

Snack

Zucchini Fries

Servings 4

2 c. zucchini, shredded

1 Tbsp. coconut flour

Salt or garlic salt

Paprika

Oregano

3 eggs

Pepper

Coconut oil

Shred up the zucchini and then set it aside for a minute. In a bowl you can beat together the eggs before carefully sifting the flour into the egg mixture and beating it all together. Next you can mix the shredded zucchini along with the pepper, spices and the salt into the egg mixture.

Warm the coconut oil in a skillet. Take the mixture and spoon it into the pan, making the fritters as big or small as you would like them as you go along. Once the fritters are done cooking, you can serve the fritters either warm or cooled down a bit.

Nutritional Facts:

Calories 98

Fat 12g

Carbs 2g

Protein 0g

Dessert

Chocolate Chip Cookies

Servings 12

1 tsp. baking soda

3 ½ c. almond flour

1 tsp. salt

1 egg

½ c. coconut oil

½ c. syrup

1 tsp. vanilla

1 ½ c. chocolate chips

Preheat oven to 375 (180C) degrees. Mix together all of your dry ingredients in a bowl. Using another bowl, whisk together the vanilla, syrup, and egg. Add this mixture to your dry ingredients and then stir.

Then add in the coconut oil and the chocolate chips, making sure to keep mixing the whole time. Place little balls of this dough on a baking sheet and flatten with the back of a spoon before placing into the oven. Allow the cookies to bake for about 15 minutes or until they turn a golden brown color. Serve these cookies right away or store for later.

Nutritional Facts

Calories 156

Fat 5g

Carbs 12g

Protein 0g

Tuesday

Breakfast

Berry Pancakes

Servings 4

1 Tbsp. coconut flour

1 c. almond flour

2 eggs

Salt

Coconut oil

½ c. unsweetened applesauce

¼ tsp. nutmeg

¼ c. water

Berries

Combine the almond flour, applesauce, coconut flour, eggs, water, nutmeg, and salt in a bowl. You will want to make sure that everything is mixed well together before continuing.

Next you can take out a skillet, add the coconut oil and gently heat on the stove. When the coconut oil has warmed up, take about ¼ of your batter and drop it into the skillet. (Test the heat of the oil, by dropping in a small amount of mixture and seeing if it fizzles, if so, it is at the right heat.)

Once the edges start to bubble a little, you can flip your pancake over and allow the other side to cook. Repeat this process so that you use up the batter. When all of the pancakes are done you can serve with fresh berries and enjoy.

Nutritional Facts

Calories 189

Fat 8g

Carbs 15g

Protein 2g

Lunch

Grilled Chicken Salad

Servings 4

½ c. carrot, grated

Sliced radishes

1 avocado sliced

3 c. arugula/rocket

¾ c. peach slices

2 grilled chicken breasts, sliced

1 tsp. cinnamon

2 Tbsp. coconut oil

1 tsp. nutmeg

Wash, peel and slice/chop all of the ingredients.

Slice up the chicken.

Heat up a skillet with the coconut oil. Once the skillet is nice and warm, place the peach slices inside and let them sauté for a few minutes before setting aside.

In a bowl, you can mix together the nutmeg, cinnamon, carrot, chicken and peaches with a small amount of coconut oil.

Arrange on top of the arugula/rocket and place the avocado, radishes and some onion around the edges.

Nutritional Facts:

Calories 112

Fat 12g

Carbs 8g

Protein 18g

Dinner

Shepherd's Pie

Servings 4

¾ lb. parsnips

Salt

1 Tbsp. olive oil

1 slice of bacon

½ lb. zucchini sliced

¼ lb. button mushrooms sliced

Coconut oil

1 celery stalk sliced

½ red onion diced

1 ¼ lb. turkey, ground or beef

2 onions diced

Oregano and Basil

Celery salt

8 egg whites (optional)

Pepper

½ c. parsley finely chopped

Preheat the oven to about 450 degrees (210C). Peel the parsnips before sprinkling with the olive oil and onion salt and setting aside.

Grill or fry the bacon until crispy and then let it cool before crumbling and setting aside.

Add the celery, mushrooms, and zucchini to the same pan the bacon was in and let it sauté for a few minutes.

Take another pan and add the coconut oil before mixing in the pepper, celery salt, oregano, basil, ground turkey, and onions. Sauté until the turkey is cooked. Combine together the vegetables and the meat into one pan before mixing thoroughly and leaving for 5 minutes to cool.

Beat 4 of the egg whites with the parsley before adding to the vegetable and meat mixture. Take the other 4 egg whites and mix with the parsnips before setting both to the side for a minute. Grease a baking dish before adding in the vegetable and meat mixture and topping with the parsnip mixture and the crumbled bacon. Bake this for around 25 minutes so the top browns and enjoy.

(You can easily use lamb or beef instead and leave out the egg whites)

Nutritional Facts

Calories 345

Fat 20g

Carbs 5g

Protein 15g

Snack

Veggie Fries

Servings 2

2 eggs

1 eggplant/brinjal/aubergine

2 c. vegan cheese

Paprika

Oregano

To start this recipe, you can get out your food processor. Turn on the oven and allow it to heat up to 450 (210C) degrees. Cut the ends of the eggplant and rinse off before shredding it through the food processor.

Mix together your shredded eggplant with the cheese, paprika, oregano and eggs before lumping it into cookie like shapes. Place the 'cookies' onto a baking sheet/tray and place into the oven to bake for about 12 minutes.

Remove from oven and flip the 'cookies' over. Place the sheet back into the oven and let the 'cookies' bake for another five minutes. Once the chips are cooked, you can take them out of the oven and cut into triangles before allowing to cool for a few hours. Enjoy right away or store in a Ziploc bag for later.

You can add a courgette or zucchini to the mix if desired.

Nutritional Facts:

Calories 85

Fat 12g

Carbs 2g

Protein 0g

Dessert

Zesty Pudding

Servings 4

1 c. coconut milk

¼ c. honey

2 tsp. cinnamon

1 tsp. orange zest

1/8 tsp. salt

¼ c. cocoa powder, unsweetened

Cayenne pepper

Raw cacao nibs

1 box silken tofu

Heat a saucepan on the stove. Combine the cinnamon and coconut milk in the saucepan and bring it all to a boil. Reduce your heat and allow this mixture to simmer for 7 minutes. Once the milk is reduced to 1/3 of a cup, take it off the heat and set aside.

In another saucepan, you can take 3 tablespoons of this mixture and combine it with the cayenne pepper, salt, cocoa powder, orange zest, and honey. Whisk these ingredients together and bring to a boil. Allow to simmer for about a minute before taking off the heat.

Pour this mixture into a blender and add the tofu before processing these ingredients until they are smooth. Transfer the mixture to a bowl and place in the fridge for a minimum of 2 hours and then serve and enjoy! Decorate with a mint leaf.

Note; It is better to grate a cinnamon stick than to use the cinnamon powder one buys in a bottle, as all that is, is effectively sawdust with no nutritional value.

Nutritional Facts

Calories 100

Fat 3g

Carbs 5g

Protein 5g

Wednesday

Breakfast

Tapioca Crepes

Servings 1

1 c. tapioca flour

1 egg

1 c. coconut milk

Salt

Any topping choice

To get started on this recipe, you will need to combine together the flour, egg, coconut milk and the salt into a bowl and then mix them completely together before setting aside.

Heat up a skillet on the stove and allow it to become warm before pouring about 1/3 of the mixture into the pan and tilting it all around to let the batter spread out evenly in the skillet.

Cook both sides until they begin to lightly brown, this will take about 3 minutes on both sides. Take the crepe off the skillet when it is done cooking. Repeat this process until all of the batter is done. Top the crepes with any ingredients you want, such as vegetables, applesauce, bacon, or cinnamon before enjoying.

Nutritional Facts:

Calories 210

Fat 12g

Carbs 6g

Protein 1g

Lunch

Crab Bisque

Servings 6

½ c. chopped onion

Olive Oil

2 Tbsp. almond flour

2 Tbsp. almond butter

2 c. chicken broth

3 c. almond milk

Salt

Cayenne pepper

1 lb. cooked crabmeat

¼ tsp. pepper

1 thyme sprig

2 garlic cloves, crushed

3 Tbsp. parsley

1 bay leaf

1 tsp. lemon juice

¼ tsp tumeric

For this recipe, you will need to get out a bowl and mix together the lemon juice and the crabmeat before setting aside.

Next, take out a skillet and warm it up on the stove with some olive oil. Once the skillet is warmed, you can place the garlic and the onion inside. Let these ingredients cook for a few minutes to become tender.

At this time, you can add in your salt and almond flour and then stir to combine. Reduce the heat a little bit before adding in the almond milk and chicken broth slowly. Add in all of your seasonings next, making sure to stir the whole time as you are reducing the heat to a low setting.

Now it is time to add in your crab meat chunks to the rest of the ingredients. Once all of the crabmeat is added, you can leave everything at a simmer and let it cook for about 15 minutes. Take out the bay leaf and thyme sprig at this time and then serve the bisque nice and warm.

Nutritional Facts:

Calories 210

Fat 10g

Carbs 3g

Protein 33g

Dinner

Beef Casserole

Servings 4

2 Tbsp. olive oil

1 onion

1 green pepper sliced

1 Carrot sliced

1 lb. ground beef

2 garlic cloves

1 can tomato sauce

Handful okra

Cumin

Chili powder

Marjoram

Heat up a skillet on the stove before adding in the oil once it is hot. Next you can add in the garlic, green pepper, okra, carrot and onion. Let these sauté for around 10 minutes so they become tender.

Then you can add in the ground beef and let everything cook until the beef is turning brown. Keep stirring regularly. This might take about 10-15 minutes. Lastly you can stir the cumin, chili powder, marjoram and tomato sauce into the mixture. Allow to simmer until meat is properly cooked. Remove this from the heat and then serve when ready.

Serve with mashed turnip and cabbage steamed with lemon and sage.

Nutritional Facts

Calories 215

Fat 10g

Carbs 3g

Protein 27g

Snack

Trail Mix

Servings 6

1 c. pumpkin seeds

1 c. roasted almonds

½ c. raisins

½ c. sunflower seeds

1 c. dried blueberries

To start this recipe, you will want to take all of the ingredients and place them into a bowl.

Toss the bowl around to combine before placing the lid on top and storing everything in a dry area. Enjoy the recipe as you like for a snack.

Nutritional Facts

Calories 102

Fat 5g

Carbs 0g

Protein 15g

Dessert

Butterscotch Ice Cream

3 Tbsp. coconut cream

1 1/3 c. almond milk

1 ripe avocado

Honey

2 Tbsp. Lucama/eggfruit

½ tsp. salt

Syrup

Nuts

Get out your blender and place all of the ingredients except the nuts and syrup inside. Pulse until smooth.

Place this mixture into your ice cream maker and follow the manufacturer instructions for how to proceed. When the ice cream is done, fold the nuts of your choice in and then enjoy with some syrup.

Nutritional Facts

Calories 276

Fat 12g

Carbs 10g

Protein 23g

Thursday

Breakfast

Vegetable Frittata

Servings 1

1 zucchini/courgette/baby marrow

1 ½ Tbsp. olive oil

½ bell pepper

1 Tbsp. thyme

½ red onion

Salt

Pepper

2 cloves of garlic

9 eggs

1 tomato chopped

Heat up the olive oil in a skillet. Once it is hot you can add the garlic, half of the salt and pepper, the thyme, onion, bell pepper and zucchini to the skillet and let them all sauté.

Reduce heat, cover skillet and cook for about 5 minutes so the vegetables can become tender. Next you can stir in the tomato. Cook everything for another 5 minutes, making sure it is uncovered.

Combine together the eggs with the rest of the salt and pepper and whisk it all together until it becomes frothy. Pour the eggs over the vegetables and stir gently. Cover and let it all simmer for 15 minutes. Invert the frittata onto your plate.

Slice it up and serve right away.

Nutritional Facts:

Calories 235

Fat 10g

Carbs 2g

Protein 19g

Lunch

Chicken Wraps

Servings 1

½ c. chopped chicken

2 Tbsp. red grapes, chopped

3 Tbsp. apples, chopped and unpeeled

2 tsp. honey

2 Tbsp. almond butter

1 lettuce leaf, romaine

For this recipe, you will want to take the time to prepare all of your ingredients. Wash off the apples and the grapes well before cutting them up into smaller pieces to use in the wrap.

Cook the chicken on the grill, which will take around 10-15 minutes. Always make sure chicken is very well cooked. Once the chicken has cooked, you can chop it into smaller pieces.

Bring out a bowl and combine together all of your ingredients except the lettuce, making sure they are well mixed. Place all of the ingredients on to the romaine lettuce leaf, wrap it up, and enjoy right away.

Nutritional Facts:

Calories 143

Fat 2g

Carbs 0g

Protein 23g

Dinner

Paleo Hamburgers

Servings 4

1 lb. ground beef

Mixed herbs

½ c. finely chopped pimento

Salt

Pepper

Coconut oil

Mix the meat, herbs and pimento together with the pepper and the salt. Take the meat and form it into about 4 evenly sized patties.

Heat up a skillet or saucepan with some coconut oil. Cook the beef to your personal preference. Serve with some of your favorite toppings.

I like to make my own tomato sauce by chopping 4 tomatoes and combining with basil, salt, ground black pepper and olive oil in a small saucepan. Bring to boil with a tablespoon of water and then reduce until a lovely chunky sauce is achieved.

Fabulous topped with guacamole (avocado, lemon juice, chopped spring onions, salt and paprika) and a side salad.

Nutritional Facts:

Calories 189

Fat 5g

Carbs 1g

Protein 15g

Snack

Blueberry Candy

Servings 4

5 c. blueberries

1 ½ tsp. ginger

4 tsp. cinnamon

¼ c. honey

2 egg whites

1 tsp. vanilla

For this recipe, you will need to start out by bringing out a bowl and whisking together the egg whites so that they become frothy. Add the vanilla and the honey to the egg whites and continue stirring until everything is combined.

Using a slotted spoon, you can add in the blueberries to this mixture. Remove a little bit of the mixture at a time and place it into another bowl that has the ginger and cinnamon inside. You will want to repeat this step until you have gotten all of the blueberries covered.

Using the same spoon, you can place your coated blueberries on a dehydrator tray. Allow the blueberries to dehydrate for at least 24 hours. About halfway through, you can turn the blueberries over to make sure that even drying is occurring.

When the blueberries are completely done drying, you can place into a container and enjoy when you are ready.

Nutritional Facts:

Calories 98

Fat 2g

Carbs 1g

Protein 5g

Dessert

Creamy Flan

Servings 12

2 c. thick cream

3 c. coconut milk

8 eggs

¼ c. honey

½ Tbsp. vanilla

¼ c. honey for caramelizing

1 Tbsp. water

Squeeze of lemon

Bring out a bowl and combine together the vanilla, ¼ c. of honey, eggs, thick cream, and coconut milk together.

Turn on the oven and let it heat up to 350 (210C) degrees. While that is heating up, you can bring out a saucepan and place the rest of the honey, the lemon juice, and the water in to heat up. Stir this mixture so that it becomes golden brown before taking off the heat.

Take out a baking/corning ware dish that is about 3 quarts along with one that is a little bigger. Pour the honey that you just caramelized into the smaller one and spread it out to cover the whole dish.

Place this dish into the larger dish before adding some water to the larger dish, no more than an inch high. Pour the blended mixture of flan into your small baking dish on top of the caramelized honey.

Place into the oven and let it cook for about 60 minutes so that it can set in the middle with a custard texture. When it is done you can take it out and place into the refrigerator for about 30 minutes before serving.

Nutritional Facts

Calories 310

Fat 20g

Carbs 15g

Protein 5g

Friday

Breakfast

Western Omelet

1 tsp. coconut oil

4 eggs

1 diced bell pepper

½ diced onion

1 diced tomato

¼ lbs. cooked ham

1 c. spinach

Salt

Pepper

Take the vegetables and wash them off before chopping them into smaller pieces, then sauté in some of the oil until tender. Next, crack the eggs into a bowl before beating them well and setting aside.

Place the coconut oil in a skillet and let it heat up before pouring half of your egg mixture into your skillet. When it has had some time to set, you can scrape off the edges and tip around the pan so the rest of the egg can get cooked.

Now you can take the ham and the vegetables and place it on half of the omelet. Continue cooking for a few more minutes so the egg can finish setting. Using your spatula, fold the egg in half and cook for two more minutes. Repeat these steps with the rest of the ingredients to get another omelet and then enjoy!

Nutritional Facts:

Calories 234

Fat 12g

Carbs 10g

Protein 20g

Lunch

Burritos

Servings 1

¼ c. refried beans

1 tortilla

¼ c. chili with beans, vegetarian

1 Tbsp. taco sauce

1 oz. feta cheese

For this easy to make recipe, you can take your tortilla and lay it down on a flat surface. Fill the tortilla with the chili, cheese, and refried beans before rolling the tortilla up nice and tightly.

Place the tortilla on to a microwavable safe plate before placing inside the microwave. Allow the tortilla to cook in the microwave for about a minute so the cheese has time to melt. After this time, you can take the tortilla out of the microwave, open it up, and then top with some salsa.

Make this tortilla your own by adding some other great toppings such as tomatoes, avocado, red onion, walnuts and lettuce without adding in a lot of extra calories and fat. Once all of the toppings have been added, you can roll the tortilla back up nice and tight again before enjoying right away.

Nutritional Facts:

Calories 297

Fat 4.7g

Carbs 30.8g

Protein 18g

Dinner

Spaghetti

Servings 4

1 Tbsp. olive oil

1 onion, chopped

2 tomatoes, chopped

1 carrot, diced

1 celery stick sliced finely

1 Tbsp. Tomato paste

Fresh parsley

1 lb. ground beef

2 garlic cloves

24 oz. kelp noodles

Heat up a skillet with some olive oil. Once the skillet has had some time to warm up, add the onion, carrot, celery and parsley and sauté until the onion is transparent, Add the tomato and sauté for another 5 mins. Season with salt and pepper. Then add the meat, tomato paste and garlic to the skillet with a cup of water and let the mixture cook until the meat is done.

Next you can add the noodles, making sure to stir it all while it is coming to a simmer. Add more water as required. Allow the ingredients to continue cooking until they are completely cooked. Serve with some vegetables of your choice and enjoy this dish right away.

I recommend serving with steamed broccoli and cabbage greens with pumpkin seeds.

Nutritional Facts:

Calories 285

Fat 2g

Carbs 0g

Protein 34g

Snack

Chocolate Cake

Servings 8

Pitted dates

3 eggs

1 c. applesauce, unsweetened

½ c. coconut oil

½ c. coconut flour

2 tsp. vanilla

½ c. cocoa powder, unsweetened

1 tsp. baking soda

½ c. brewed coffee

½ tsp. sea salt

Warm up your oven to 350 (210C) degrees. While the oven is warming up, you will need to bring out your food processor and place the dates inside. Pulse these dates for a couple of minutes so that they are completely pureed.

At this time, you can add the applesauce to the food processor and continue pulsing so that you get a nice puree. Next, take this fruit puree and add it to a bowl and mix with the brewed coffee, coconut oil, vanilla and eggs. Mix these ingredients well.

Taking out another bowl and combine the dry ingredients. Slowly combine the wet ingredients together with the dry ingredients until you are left with a smooth batter.

Pour this batter into a prepared tin, making sure to smooth it down with a spatula before placing into the oven to bake. Bake the cake for about 30 minutes or until it is done. Give it a few minutes to cool down before enjoying.

Nutritional Facts:

Calories 215

Fat 20g

Carbs 3g

Protein 2g

Dessert

Grilled Bananas

Servings 2

1 tsp. cinnamon

2 bananas with peels

Coconut oil

You can brush the quartered bananas with some coconut oil and sprinkle the cinnamon on for taste.

Place the bananas on the grill and let them cook for about 4 minutes. Flip them over and grill for another 4 minutes.

Take off the grill and peel and serve the bananas right away.

Nutritional Facts:

Calories 100

Fat 5g

Carbs 5g

Protein 10g

Saturday

Breakfast

Zucchini Muffins

Servings 12

½ c. coconut flour

1 c. almond flour

2 tsp. baking soda

½ c. tapioca flour

1 tsp. salt

1 Tbsp. allspice

1 Tbsp. cinnamon

1 c. pitted dates

3 eggs

3 bananas

1 tsp. vinegar, apple cider

5 oz. frozen berries

¼ c. coconut oil

¾ c. almonds

¾ c. zucchini

Give your berries some time to thaw out before beginning this recipe. While the berries are thawing out, you can turn on the oven and let it warm up to 350 (210C) degrees.

Next, take out a bowl and combine together the allspice, cinnamon, salt, baking soda, tapioca flour, coconut flour, and the almond flour. Bring out your food processor and combine together the oil, vinegar, eggs, bananas, and dates before transferring to another bowl and stirring to combine with the other ingredients.

Slowly fold in the almonds, zucchini, and berries next before spooning this mixture into your muffin tin and placing into the oven. Allow the muffins to bake for about 20 minutes or until they are completely done.

Nutritional Facts:

Calories 190

Fat 5g

Carbs 23g

Protein 2g

Lunch

Chicken Fajitas

3 minced garlic cloves

1 tsp. oregano

1 tsp. cumin

1 tsp. chili powder

1 lb. chicken breast fillet

1 tsp. salt

1 Tbsp. coconut oil

2 sliced red bell peppers

½ sliced red onion

Juice from 1 lemon

Juice from 1 lime

Guacamole (avocado mashed with grated onion and paprika)

2 heads of lettuce

1 jar salsa

Combine together the salt, chili powder, oregano, cumin, and garlic in a bowl. Toss the chicken in with this mixture so that it can become coated on all sides and then set aside.

Next, heat up a pan with the coconut oil. When it is warmed up, you can sauté the onion for about 3 minutes before adding in the chicken and letting it all cook for another 10 minutes so that the chicken is cooked through. Right before the chicken finishes, you can add in the lime juice, lemon juice, and red peppers.

Cook everything for another 3 minutes. Serve everything over the lettuce and top with some salsa and guacamole before enjoying.

Nutritional Facts:

Calories 285

Fat 10g

Carbs 22g

Protein 32g

Dinner

Lime and Dill Crab

Servings 4

2 Dungeness crabs

1 tsp. paprika

Juice from 1 lime

2 tsp. chopped dill

Heat up a pot full of water so that the water starts to boil. Once the water starts boiling, drop the crabs in and let them cook for about 8 minutes.

After that time, you can take the crabs out of the water and put them under some cold water so they become easy to handle. When the crab has cooled down, crack the shells and take the meat out before drizzling on the dill, paprika, and lime juice. Serve this dish with some lime wedges and enjoy.

Wonderful with a watercress, avocado, kiwi fruit and grapefruit salad.

Nutritional Facts:

Calories 218

Fat 5g

Carbs 12g

Protein 23g

Snack

Salmon Poppers

Servings 10

1 head endive

½ minced red onion

½ a cucumber peeled and sliced

5 bottled artichoke hearts

4 oz. salmon, smoked

Salt

Pepper

½ sliced avocado

Olive oil

Balsamic vinegar

Take your endive leaves and wash them off before separating. Place the leaves on a clean surface before topping with the avocado, artichokes, cucumber, red onion, and smoked salmon. Add a little ground black pepper and sea salt to your taste before drizzling on the olive oil. Mixed with balsamic vinegar. Once everything is how you like it, serve right away.

Nutritional Facts:

Calories 118

Fat 8g

Carbs 14g

Protein 11g

Dessert

Almond Macaroons

Servings 12

1/8 tsp. cinnamon

1 ¼ c. almonds

2 beaten egg whites

1 tsp. lemon zest

1 tsp. lemon juice

¼ c. honey

Turn on the oven and let it preheat to 250 (120C) degrees. While the oven is heating up, you can grind up the almonds coarsely before setting aside. Mix together the lemon zest and cinnamon in a bowl.

Beat your egg whites before adding them in to the cinnamon mixture along with the lemon juice and honey. Stir all of these together vigorously so that they are blended through. Next, take out a baking sheet and line it with some greaseproof paper.

Use a small scoop to place little portions of this batter on the baking sheet before placing it into the oven. Bake these macaroons for about 30 minutes or until done. Give them a few minutes to cool down before enjoying!

Nutritional Facts:

Calories 245

Fat 5g

Carbs 24g

Protein 1g

Sunday

Breakfast

Pumpkin Muffins

Servings 12

¾ c. pumpkin or butternut, cooked

1 ½ c. almond flour

3 eggs

1 tsp. baking soda

1 tsp. baking powder

½ tsp. cinnamon

1/8 tsp. salt

1 ½ tsp. all spice

¼ c. honey

1 Tbsp. almonds, sliced

2 tsp. butter, almond

Turn the oven on to 350 (170C) degrees to warm up. While the oven is warming up, you can take a muffin tin and coat it with some coconut oil. Mix together all of the ingredients in a bowl until they are well combined before pouring into your prepared muffin tins and placing into the oven.

Bake the muffins for about 25 minutes in the middle of the oven before taking them out and enjoying!

Nutritional Facts:

Calories 213

Fat 12g

Carbs 33g

Protein 0g

Lunch

Grilled Veggies

Servings 4

Juice from 1 lime

¾ lb. shrimp

1 sliced zucchini/baby marrow/courgette

Pepper

1 red onion sliced thickly

1 sliced summer squash, yellow

1 sliced bell pepper, red

1 sliced bell pepper, green

3 Tbsp. olive oil

4 minced garlic gloves, skewers

Prepare shrimp by peeling and washing before placing into a bowl. Add the pepper and the lime juice to the bowl and set to the side for about five minutes. While the shrimp is soaking, you can take your vegetables and wash and chop them up.

Turn on the grill at this time so that it has time to warm up. Add your garlic, olive oil, and vegetables to the bowl with the shrimp and toss to combine. Place the shrimp and the veggies onto the skewers and then place on the grill to cook. After everything is well cooked, you can take off the grill and enjoy.

Nutritional Facts

Calories 95

Fat 4g

Carbs 4g

Protein 22g

Dinner

Vegetable And Turkey Meatballs

Servings 4

2 carrots

1 lb. ground chicken

1 bell pepper, green

5 mushrooms

Handful curly leaf parsley

1 clove garlic

½ onion

2 tsp. garlic salt

½ tsp. pepper

2 Tbsp. Italian seasoning (Oregano, Basil, Sage, Marjoram)

1 egg

Preheat the oven so that it can warm up to 350F (160C) degrees. While the oven is heating up, you can combine together the seasonings, garlic, onion, mushrooms, bell pepper, and carrots to your food processor.

Let them blend so they become well chopped up. Empty these ingredients into a bowl before adding the ground chicken and egg. Mix everything together well. When the ingredients are mixed, you can form them into meatballs before placing onto a baking sheet and placing into the oven.

The meat balls can also be placed in a casserole dish with a small amount of oil and water to cook.

Allow the meatballs to bake for 25 minutes before serving.

Nutritional Facts:

Calories 222

Fat 9g

Carbs 14g

Protein 25g

Snack

Deviled Eggs With Guacamole

Servings 4

1 avocado

4 hard-boiled eggs

2 tsp. Tabasco sauce or chili sauce

Salt

Chopped spring onions

1 tsp. lemon juice

Pepper

To start this recipe, hard-boil the eggs. When that is done, you can peel them before cutting in half length wise. Spoon out the yolks from the eggs into a bowl before mashing them together with the lemon juice, hot sauce, and avocado. Stir in the spring onions.

Make sure to season with a little bit of pepper and salt to taste. Once the mixture is done, you can refill your eggs with it and then serve.

Nutritional Facts:

Calories 88

Fat 2g

Carbs 6g

Protein 11g

Dessert

Brownies

Servings 12

3 c. almond flour

2 eggs

¾ c. honey

¼ c. coconut oil

½ c. unsweetened cocoa powder

1 tsp. ginger

1 tsp. nutmeg

¼ tsp. salt

Preheat the oven to 350F (160C) degrees. While the oven is heating up, you can use the coconut oil to grease up your baking pan. Next, take out a saucepan and warm both the oil and the honey inside it before setting aside. Sift together the spices, cocoa powder, salt and flour into a bowl.

In another bowl you can stir together the vanilla, ginger, eggs and the honey before adding this into the flour mixture. Make sure to stir until it becomes well blended. Transfer this mixture to a pan and let it bake for about 25 minutes or until done. Give it a few minutes to cool down before enjoying.

Nutritional Facts:

Calories 246

Fat 15g

Carbs 25g

Protein 1g

FINAL WORD ON FOOD

Wow, I bet you didn't expect to see some of those great meal choices when you heard the word paleo? Now, let me ask you a question. How many of you have been eating some of these great dishes in the past? Well if you have then you have already tried the paleo diet.

As you can see going paleo doesn't mean eating rice cake and drinking protein shakes. It is about eating real food but doing it in a different way. Now that you have seen what is on the paleo diet why not try it for a week and see how you feel and what it does for you.

What About Exercise?

Exercise, yuck!

I know that is what you are thinking. I only exercise if a balls are involved – no, don't even go there - and with my workload and the British weather, how often can I really get onto the tennis court. I mean yeah I go out and walk but I don't have the time to go to the gym, wait for a machine to come available, figure out how to work the stupid thing and then do a few reps before I am worn out and want sit down with an ice pack. I know exercise is important but isn't there a better way and also a less expensive way than the gym?

Well when it comes to exercise on the Paleo diet you are not required to be lifting heavy weights, running miles upon miles, hitting the heavy bays or all of the other exercises that you are dreading.

No, you don't have to join a gym or spend thousands of dollars on a personal coach. When it comes to exercise on the Paleo diet it is focused on your natural movements. When you look at the basis of the Paleo diet you are going back to the basics of eating and lifestyle. So with that being said the same is true for exercise.

When you exercise on the Paleo diet it should be used to compliment your healthy diet and lifestyle. When you start exercising on the Paleo diet you are working to improve your immune system, lower your risks for diabetes, strokes, cancer, and a slew of other health issues that come on with age.

When you get regular exercise you begin to feel better. The positivity inducing hormones start to flow. You reduce stress and start to really feel the beneficial effects of the Paleo diet. You will start to gain lean muscle tone and maybe a sexy physique that will make your lover shiver. Now who doesn't want that?

The approach to exercise in the Paleo diet allows your body to take full advantage of physical activity while avoiding any negative effects or forcing you to move your body in ways that you can't or that it wasn't originally designed to move in.

Paleo exercise focuses on natural movements

What is involved, you ask?

Now doctors will tell you that you need to get a lot of cardio workouts into your diet plan. Well on Paleo we don't recommend this. We feel that too much cardio is bad for the body and doesn't give you the desired result that you are looking for.

When you have too much cardio your body goes into what we like to call the "fight or flight" mode. It also increases the possibility of inflammation and damage to your body and joints.

When you are on a high carb diet doing cardio on a long term basis, the result will be a rise in your insulin levels which can cause damage to many parts of your body. Unlike some exercise programs, the Paleo exercise plan stresses rest and recovery as the main principal to its workout routine. This mindset will help your body to feel strong and energized compared to sore and exhausted.

When you exercise you need to know your body's limits. You never want to feel as if you are torturing your body into doing something. When you do that you are defeating the purpose. No matter what diet plan you decide to try you, never want to overdo exercise. When you overdo exercise you are defeating the purpose of what exercise is supposed to do for you.

The ultimate goal of exercise is to help strengthen your body and to maintain your health. When you overdo exercise or force yourself to do something that you are not ready to do, then you are being counterproductive. You are actually causing more damage to your body than doing good.

With this being said you are probably confused on what exactly Paleo exercise is. Well it is a very flexible workout routine. Each exercise routine is tailored to each individual person just as the food part of the diet is flexible for each individual person.

You just need to know how it works for you.

NATURAL MOVEMENTS

Now when you look at the Paleo diet, you now know we are looking back at how the cavemen lived their lives. The caveman didn't have gyms, elliptical training machines, thy masters, weights, swimming pools, or the dvd players to watch Tae bo. With this being said you are going to be working with a narrow range of movements.

When you move your body on machines you are moving your body in an unnatural way. Yes I know they tell you that these machines are on the cutting edge of science and "simulate" human movements, but why do you need them when you naturally move with human movements already. When you exercise in the Paleo style you are only working on a range of thirteen fundamental movements.

These thirteen fundamental movements have been broken down into these three categories. Manipulative, combative, locomotive.

Manipulative – **This series of movements refer to moving objects around. When you move things around you are working on many different parts of the body. You are working with your hands, arms, legs, feet, back. Think of this back in the age of the caveman. The caveman was constantly on the move. Either for shelter, survival from the weather, food supplies, water supplies or just to explore the world in which they inhabited.**

The same is true today. Of course we are not moving to stay away from predators or searching for food. In our modern culture we are actually getting away from this fundamental movement. We sit in our cars as we drive to and from where we need to go to. We sit in chairs staring at computer screens all day doing mindless tasks. When we get home we are tired so we sit down in a chair or on a couch and watch television or listen to the radio or surf the net until it is time to go to bed. Then when we wake up we get up and repeat the same process all over again.

Think of how many thing we do however, that do involve movement: pushing a trolley, a lawnmower, a vacuum cleaner or sweeping. Cleaning the car, digging in the garden, moving furniture. All these qualify as manipulative and they are things we already do every day. Doing chores can be doing exercise and if those chores are outdoors even better.

The message is be more active, do things about the home, volunteer to help others and get a double whammy of exercise and the feel good factor of achieving something.

Combative – **This is another natural movement that we have gotten away from. In the past our caveman ancestors were in a constant state of combativeness. At a single instant their lives could be lost.**

When you are in a combative state you are alert and aware of your surroundings. In today's culture we are in a general state of relaxation. Yes, we are a little like zombies tuned into our devices, but not into our surroundings. The fear that a wild animal or other danger coming into our lives is limited. The odds of a wild bear or a mountain lion waling into your house is slim to none. So with this danger eliminated we no longer feel the need to be in a combative state. Yes, we may fear muggers and motorists when we cross the road, but in general we are far too complacent about our relative safety.

When our caveman brothers and sisters were around they were constantly in a state of awareness. They had to know what was coming, how many were coming and what their intentions were. Then when a threat did pose itself they were able to react within a moment's notice.

When you are moving in a combative way you are using the muscles in your back, arms and legs. Your adrenalin is pumping through your body, your blood pressure rises and blood flows through your body at an accelerated rate.

When this happened you start to burn calories, fats and other stored resources in the body. Also, your body begins to build muscle tone and create antibodies that will be used to protect it from damage from any threat that may come your way.

Being in a combative mode is good for many reasons. When you add stress to that mix you are being counterproductive but that can easily be relieved once you have a handle on the situation.

So as a modern man or woman you should try to work yourself up physically like the caveman did. Now I am not saying put yourself in a dangerous situation, but start by working your body up so that your adrenalin levels rise, your heart begins to pump blood and you start to take advantage of the physical effects the cavemen enjoyed.

How do you do this? Love relationships and flirting. Sex. Sports where you have to be alert and think fast i.e. tennis, football, rugby, table tennis, cycling, extreme sports, skateboarding, rollerblading, competitive swimming and running, swimming in the sea, cross country, hunting etc. Looking after children also qualifies as you have to be very alert with kiddies around. As you can see, it is easy to find activities to engage in which are combative.

Locomotive

In other words get your butt off the couch, step away from the computer, put down your cell phone and get moving. One major factor in the health and wellbeing of the cavemen was that they were constantly moving. They didn't have the luxury of Lay-Z-Boy recliners or heated seats in high end automobiles. The caveman was up from dawn looking for food, staking out land for shelter and trying to avoid being eaten by whatever they were hunting.

When your body is in a constant state of movement you don't have time to sit and let fat build up in your body. When you are constantly moving you are constantly burning fat and calories.

We live in a got-to-have-it-now society. The problem is that the way we get it now is by sitting down and pushing a button. And it has only gotten worse. Back in the 1980's when I was growing up we had to get up and change the channel on the television. There was a little wooden colored box that had an a / b switch on it. Then there were six toggle switches. The top toggle switches were 1 – 6 and the bottom toggle switches were 7 – 12. These were the channels we had growing up. And when something was on that we didn't want to watch we had to walk up to the box and start flipping switches. We went to places called libraries and had to Photostat articles we needed for school; if in doubt we had to ask grandparents and older relatives for their recollection of world events – the way I am talking younger readers may think the 80's were the caveman era. Bottom line is, in the past, information, food, advice, social life, music etc. was all harder to come by and you needed to get out and about to access these things.

Now a days we sit in chairs and click a single button and flip through over 500 channels. Yes, even today there is nothing on and what is on, is remade over and over again with a different name, but that is a topic for another book or rant on a blog post. Anyway, the point I am trying to get across is that we have become a society that doesn't get off our butts anymore and do anything: simple.

Let's take a look at a typical day in a life of an average person.

Wake up – I don't know about you but I get up about eight in the morning. Some people get up and have to go to a job so they may have to get up about five or six in the morning. Me, I get up and walk a few feet to my computer and sit back down. So as you can see there is really no physical activity here.

Shower – After waking up most people head to the shower. The shower usually lasts about five to ten minutes. After showering they get dressed and go get something to eat.

Breakfast – Breakfast is what we call the most important meal of the day. Why is that? Well because it is what gives us the energy we need to get our morning started and the energy to get through the rest of the day. Well the problem in today's modern society is that we don't eat breakfast or at least a full breakfast. We usually grab a piece of toast, beagle, and cup of strong coffee and run out the door.

Well the problem with this is that it is a high carb breakfast. Why is that bad? It is bad because we are not active enough in the morning to burn off those carbs. We generally eat it in our cars where we are sitting down and then we get to our jobs where we are sitting down. So those carbs from that little breakfast just sit there turning to glucose which in turn turns to fat.

When eating breakfast you should eat enough food that you are filled up but not full. You want to eat healthy foods like eggs, bacon, haddock, kipper, fruit and juice. The idea is to give yourself enough food to get the energy you need and not eat the foods that will turn to glucose, sugar, fat and all the other stuff that we don't want. Also, you want to make sure not to eat too much that you feel groggy and want to go back to bed.

Commute – Okay after breakfast you get in your car, this commute typically for most people is twenty to forty minutes. The bad thing about this, is that this is the time of the day where you are at your most rested and your body is conditioned to take in what it needs to take in and release what it needs to release. If you don't take advantage of this time your body will start to shut down and not take advantage of the fat burning period that it is ready for. This is why walking to work or having to walk a significant distance from bus stop/train to work or cycling to work can really help you burn calories.

Work – After your commute you will arrive at work. When you get to work you usually grab a doughnut or some other carb filled food that someone was so kind to pick up for everyone while on their way into the office. Eating this carb filled food is not a good idea. Since you are not in a position to work it off it will sit in your gut and convert to sugar and fat.

While at work you sit in front of a computer screen for about three hours before your first break. During this time everything that you ate has turned into glucose and making its way into sugar and fat. When you start your break you probably feel hungry so instead of going and getting something healthy to eat you go in search of those three hour old doughnuts that were brought into work. If you can't find them then you go in search of another unhealthy alternative.

As you go through your day, your energy level gets lower and lower. You attribute it to stress at work or the lack of motivation in your job. The cold hard fact is that it has nothing to do with your job. It is that doughnut or other unhealthy food choice you made about eight hours earlier.

So, in an attempt to pick yourself up you get back into your car and drive with a few of your coworkers to the nearest Starbucks/Nero/McDonalds/Cafe Rouge or some bar for a few drinks and more carbo and sugar loaded foods. Now this is just adding insult to injury

THE BAR –

When you go to a bar to have a few drinks you are just adding carbs, sugars and calories to your already tired body. Now I am not a prude or someone who has never sat in a bar before, so I am not condemning it I am just saying we shouldn't do it.

Now while you are sitting there socializing with your coworkers and friends you take a sip of beer or wine, then another and another. Now I am not going to give you a drinking and driving speech, I am just saying that every time you take a sip of beer or other alcoholic beverage you are adding unwanted non-paleo items to your body.

HOME

After you had a few at the bar you safely get in your car and drive home. If you are not safe to drive don't. You won't be worrying about Paleo if you are dead or in jail. Once you get home you kick off your shoes, give your hobby a kiss. You sit on the couch and turn on the television.

DINNER

After relaxing for a few minutes you usually have dinner. Now depending on your day you may have gotten something at the bar or picked up something from a takeout restaurant or you are eating leftovers or even a freshly cooked meal. No matter which one, it is it is probably a very large meal. The meal may be heavy with grease, carbs, calories, salt, sugar and all the great tasting stuff we deserve after a long day's work. The problem is that you are starting to shut down for the day. This is the type of meal that you should have had in the morning. Now I know what you are going to say, you don't want to have such a heavy meal in the morning. Well I agree with you.

After eating your dinner you clean up the dishes and head over to the couch and let your food digest. Well again, this is something that you don't want to do. You should get up and do some type of physical activity. I know what you are going to tell me, I don't feel like doing anything physical. Well I know because you are probably not eating Paleo.

You sit in front of the television and watch your favorite program. Then you either fall asleep on the couch or drag your body up the stairs and go to bed.

You wake up the next morning and repeat the entire process again.

Now how close was I in explaining a typical day? Now of course each person is different but in today's society this is the typical routine.

So how is one to combat this issue? Well like stated before I went into my little story, you need to get up and start moving. If you just get up and do limited exercise on a regular basis you will start to see results.

Instead of sitting in front of your computer until your break time, why not get up and take a quick walk around the office. Go to the bathroom or talk to someone in the hall. I know that some bosses are very strict in what they want you to do and how you are supposed to do it but this is your health we are talking about.

When working out in the Paleo method you want to keep your body moving as much as possible. Reflect back on these three aspects of movement and try to incorporate them into your life as much as possible.

OVERALL STRENGTH AND CONDITIONING

When starting, you want to do what is known as cross-fit training. The cross-fit training is the most popular of the Paleo fitness training cycles. Cross-fit training builds and works on the overall fitness and targets your overall wellbeing by incorporating your own body weight in the workout. Back in the days of cavemen, they used their own body weight to strengthen their bodies. They also did what was known as Olympic lifting. You can use this Olympic training and scale the programs to meet your own fitness levels.

When it comes to cross-fit training it focuses on slow movements, compound lifting exercises and bodyweight training to build strength. At more advanced levels, cross-fit also incorporates occasional sprinting and high intensity training. Cross-fit focuses on functional strengths and not cardio workouts.

Working out on the Paleo diet should never feel like you are doing hard work. Those on the Paleo diet feel that exercise should be fun and accommodating. If you are working out just to work out because you were told that you need to work out because you are required to, then you are working out for the wrong reasons.

POWERLIFTING

Now while the cross-fit approach to exercise is great they only focus on overall conditioning. There will be times where you just want to focus on a specific part of your body. This is where the powerlifting aspect of the Paleo exercise routine comes into play.

Powerlifting is designed to focus on increasing your muscle mass. Now if you are a male you may be very interested in this aspect of the Paleo exercise routine. If you are a woman you may not be as interested.

When it comes to powerlifting you are dealing with three basic common features. These are compound lifts over isolation exercise, free weights over machines and lifting heavier weights over fewer reps.

COMPOUND LIFTS

Compound lifts builds strength more efficiently than isolation exercises. By doing compound lifts you are working more muscle groups in the body with each exercise.

The first type of compound lift is known as a squat. The second compound list is called a deadlift. From there we will go into bench pressing and then rows. From there we will go to the dreaded chin-ups or pull-ups. I hated those as a child. Swinging from the jungle gym all the kids laughing at you. Well I digress.

From those we move on to military press / overhead presses. I am not going to go into detail about these particular lifts but you can Google them and find out more about how they are done. This is a book on Paleo not exercising.

FREE WEIGHTS

When you work with free weights you are getting more of a return than if you were to work out on many different machines at the gym. When you work out on machines at the gym you are not working your stabilizing muscles and are causing damage to your body by forcing it into unnatural positions.

LIFTING HEAVIER WEIGHTS OVER FEWER REPS

Lifting heavier weights over a shorter rep period helps build more muscles mass. You want to plan your lifting routine on a 5 x 5 system. The 5 x 5 system states that you do 5 reps of 5 lifts each. So for example you lift the weight from an extended position to your chest and down again. This is equal to one rep. What you want to do is repeat this process five times. After the fifth time you want to rest for a moment or two with your arm in the extended position. Another thing you can do is when your first arm is down is to repeat the process with your other arm. You will want to repeat this process 5 times with each arm to get the best results.

GO AT YOUR OWN PACE

When you get into powerlifting you want to go at your own pace. If you start to research powerlifting you will see Photoshop enhanced photos of men and women who look so strong they should be in the next He-man cartoon. When you get into powerlifting you don't want to overdo it. This is true with any exercise program.

You want to go at your own pace and temper your results. You are not going to get the results that you want by over working your body. When you over work your body you will be prone to strain and injury. Go at your own pace and don't feel pressured by anyone physically, verbally or by imagery of the dream body you want to have.

Each person is different and your results will vary. You can be a person that lifts weights for five minutes a day and bulk up like the hulk or you can be someone who exercises on a daily basis and doesn't see any type of results.

Don't stress out about it. Just go with the flow and allow your body to work naturally. This is the best way to get results in any exercise program you choose to try.

REST AND RECOVERY

One of the main things that you will find when you do more in-depth research into exercise on the Paleo diet, is that all the exercise will emphasize rest and recovery. It is very important to work your body as well as rest your body. As in life as well as money there are two sides to every coin. You have to work to see results but you need to let the results happen.

Look at it in the context of a car. You like to drive your car but sooner or later you will need to pull over to the side of the road and let it cool off and recharge. The same goes for your body when it comes to exercise. You can only do so much before it tells you okay shut me off I am tired and need to cool off. No matter how much you push yourself or your car, it will still tell you that and the more you push it the less performance you will get until you push it so far that no matter what you do it won't go any further.

So make sure to implement rest. Rest between reps, between exercise activity and after your exercise session. There is nothing worse than pushing your body beyond its limits. So rest and recover.

MOVEMENTS THAT FIT YOUR LIFESTYLE

When working with exercises, you don't want to stop. What I mean by this, is after you go to the gym and do your workout you want to keep moving. You want to go to the grocery store, you want to chase after your kids and you want to just stroll around the park. What you don't want to do is go home and sit on the couch for the remainder of the day watching reruns of Star Trek while scarfing down a bag of potato chips with a beer chaser.

You want to keep the momentum that you built up going. When you start you don't want to just quit and lie down and go to sleep. You want to keep the process going until the last possible minute. Once you have completed your daily activities and you are approaching your daily shut down session then you can sit in front of the TV. Don't think because you went to the gym you are off the hook for the rest of the day and you can just lay back and chill. No, you just got started. So get up, get moving and live your life.

CONCLUDING YOUR WORKOUTS

The last thing that I have to say about workouts is this, just get up and do it. You don't have to spend thousands of dollars on gym memberships or coaching programs. You just need to look at what exercises you like to do and go and do them. If you like playing basketball then go and play basketball. If you enjoy jogging go for a jog. If you want specific exercises for Paleo you can Google them or just follow the advice listed above. Just remember to not overdo it and always relax and recover for best results.

Eating Out

Eating out can be a fun and enjoyable experience. You go out to a restaurant with your friends and have a few drinks, have a few laughs and just de-stress from a long work day or even a long work week. Maybe you are on vacation and you obviously can't go home and cook or you are somewhere where you can't cook and let's face it you don't want to cook on vacation. So what are you going to do?

Well most of us have a private chief that travels with us everywhere we go. Didn't you get one when you moved out of your parent's house? Oh wait, those were your parents. Well if you don't travel with mom and dad or live with them in your thirties it will be your responsibility to figure out how and what to eat when you go out.

Now in general this isn't a real issue. It does become an issue when you are on a special diet or if you have decided to go Paleo.

Now I know there are pizza restaurants, Greek restaurants, Italian restaurants, Mexican restaurants and the list goes on and on and on. But let me ask you. When was the last time you saw a Paleo restaurant?

Well the truth is that there are no strictly Paleo restaurants. Now this is another great marketing idea. I already gave you the one for the frozen Paleo dinners. Now I just gave you the idea for the Paleo restaurant. Just remember to send me my royalty check each month.

Okay, seriously. When it comes to eating Paleo it is very hard to get Paleo food at a restaurant. So what are you to do? Well you can't stay home and live a sheltered life every time you want to eat something. You have to socialize with friends so are you going to eat dinner before you go out and sit there staring at everyone else eating making everyone uncomfortable? I would hope not.

In this section I am going to give you some tips that you can use when going out to eat. You can take these and expand on them to fit them into your lifestyle. If you have other tips that you think would fit in please jot them down and share them with others.

TIP #1 – DECIDE ON WHAT YOU ARE GOING TO ORDER BEFORE YOU GO OUT

We live in a wonderful world where information is just a fingertip away. Before we had the Internet we had to use the telephone and call the restaurant. We then got some rude hostess who didn't really like her job so she would be short with you. Now with the advent of modern technology you can go to the restaurant's web site and look up their menu.

You can take your time and review everything that is listed. You can look at your approved and not approved food lists when it comes to Paleo and decide if it is something that you want to eat or not. Then when you get to the restaurant you can look cool by sitting there knowing what you want to order. More and more restaurants now often gluten free options and so it is worth researching online.

TIP #2 – EAT BEFORE YOU GO OUT

Now this sounds like a double negative. Why in the world would you eat something if you were going to go out to eat? Well there are many reasons why you would want to eat before you go to the restaurant.

First off, if you are on the Paleo diet you can eat something Paleo before you get to the restaurant. Doing this will keep you from ordering something that isn't Paleo. Also, if you eat something before you go out you curb your appetite which makes you less hungry. If you are not real hungry when you go out you can order something light like a salad, soup or a fruit salad.

Also, eating before you go out ensures that you won't be hungry if there is very little on the menu that you can eat.

If you think about it Paleo is meat and veg – most restaurants offer salads (tick) and most have meat, fish, seafood and chicken dishes (tick). All you have to do is order a side potion of veg or a salad, chose which meat to go for and ask the waiter to leave off the fries or cheesy sauce.

Many places do all day breakfasts and eggs, bacon, mushrooms and tomatoes are allowed on Paleo.

TIP #3 –PICK THE RESTAURANT

When going out try to pick the restaurant. When you pick the restaurant you have control over what is served. If you recall, some of the recipes in the previous chapter have steak, chicken and seafood. When going out you want to stick to these types of restaurants.

Steak houses are a great choice as a lot of people love steak. BBQ joints are great as well. Sushi Bars are super trendy and easy in which to choose Paleo. Eating Italian is hard due to all the pizza and pasta having wheat and cheese, but my local Italian now has an eggplant vegan dish, a seafood salad and a chicken salad which are Paleo. Thai food often uses coconut milk instead of diary which is handy. Japanese restaurants are very Paleo friendly as well. And why not enjoy a curry without the rice?

I am sure in your area there are lots of places that serve something that everyone in your group likes. And if not bring them somewhere they can experience Paleo for themselves. Who knows, you might convert them over without even knowing it.

TIP #4 – STICK TO NATIONAL CHAINS

When you stick to national chains with a standardized menu, they are bound to have foods that will satisfy those on the Paleo diet and who are not.

When going to these restaurants make sure that you stay away from dishes that have sauces or other items that may contain sugars or non Paleo additives. Breading is also a concern when going to these places. In some cases the cooks can remove these items and in some situations they can't. Just ask questions and make sure that you can do what is needed to stay Paleo.

TIP #5 – STAY AWAY FROM CERTAIN RESTAURAUNTS

Now there are just some places you just can't go because they don't have anything you can eat. Now this doesn't mean if your friends go there you have to stay home and do laundry and sulk. You can go to these places but just don't eat. Now this can be awkward depending on the situation but if your friends just like the atmosphere there and you want to hang out then show up after they have eaten or meet up with them later at another location.

TIP #6 – ASK QUESTIONS ABOUT THE MENU

When you go out it is a common practice not to piss off the person handling your food. While this is true, you are also the one paying or at least eating the meal. So when you get to the restaurant don't be afraid to ask questions. Just be polite to your host and make sure that your questions are clear and to the point. If the host doesn't know the answer be polite and ask them to find out for you.

More and more people are intolerant/allergic to one thing or another and I often hear other customers asking questions now days. You can ring up at a quiet time to get the information, so at least when you get there at 7pm when it's crowded and noisy, you don't have to get into a long discussion then.

In most situations the host is knowledgeable about the menu. They are aware of how things are prepared and what can be substituted and what cannot. Just don't be afraid to ask a question as you may be paying for the meal in one way or another.

TIP #7 – STATE YOU ARE ALLERGIC TO GLUTEN

Now you may laugh when you hear this but it is true. There are cases where people are allergic to gluten. If you are one such person it is important to tell your server, host or whomever takes your order to note that you are allergic.

We are in a sue me state mentality and if someone were to get ill in a restaurant after stating that they were allergic to something and then were served it, that person could sue that restaurant. So if you are allergic tell your server and make sure that it is written down. Have the server show you that they wrote it down. If there is a problem you want to note the chain in which it happened. If it was never written down then it is the servers fault or his word against yours type situation. If he did write it down it is between the cook and the server.

The bottom line is making sure to tell your server and make sure to double and triple check to ensure that your food is safe for you to eat.

TIP #8 – DOES IT COME WITH BREADING?

When ordering your food you want to ask if it comes with breading. Breading is a no no when it comes to Paleo. If it comes breaded ask if they can remove the breading. If the breading can't be removed ask for an alternative to the main meat.

TIP #9 – TELL THEM YOU DON'T LIKE IT OR ARE ALLERGIC

We kind of touched on this when we talked about saying you were allergic to gluten earlier in the list. This is more of a specific allergy. If there is something that you can't eat, it is easier to tell them that you are allergic then to try to tell them you are on a Paleo diet. Now this can backfire if it's something that you need to live on or no one on the planet is allergic to. But if you can work it out to make them believe you are allergic then it is all the better for you.

TIP #10 –PRESCRIBED DIET ON DOCTOR'S ORDERS

Now this is more convincing than saying you are allergic to something. With the onset of obesity, high blood pressure, food allergies and countless other conditions doctors are restricting the diets of many of their patients.

When going into a restaurant tell your server that you are on a special diet and see if they have a special diet menu or section. On many menus they have charts and coded symbols that tell you if it is good or falls within a special diet guidelines. The worse thing that can happen is that you can't eat anything and will have to go to another restaurant or eat something more filling when you get home.

TIP #11 – ASK ABOUT THE COOKING OIL

Now this may seem like a strange request but it is the main reason why people have the issues that they do when they go out. When I go out I see tons of options for shrimp, chicken or meat. I mean what else is there. The problem arises with what the food is cooked in. In most restaurants the food is fried – well that is why it tastes nice right? The problem with fried food is that they fry it in the wrong oil. So what oil do they fry it in? Well 99% of the world's restaurants fry their foods in corn, vegetable or canola oil. You want to have your food cooked in olive oil if at all possible. Now olive oil is usually available in most restaurants so getting it shouldn't be an issue you may just have to ask for it.

TIP #12 –BEWARE OF ADDED SUGAR IN YOUR FOODS

Sugar is a main ingredient in many items we eat when dining out. There are sugars in sauces, syrups and in other products that are used during the cooking process. Now being a waiter you may not know every ingredient that is used in the cooking process. Heck, the chef might not even know. Most restaurants get a lot of prepackaged goods sent in, not everything is even made in the kitchen, and it is merely heated up.

Since all of these items are standardized for that particular restaurant those behind the scenes may not even think about what is in the food they just add heat and serve. So if at all possible ask if there are any added items in the food that the common employee may not know about. If it a real concern for you, you can go and contact the corporate offices of the restaurant and ask for a breakdown of what is in their food since you like their company but are restrictive on the diet.

TIP #13 – ASK THE CHEF

Waiters are waiters and chefs are chefs. You are not expected as a waiter to know everything that goes on in the job of everyone else in the restaurant. This includes the cooks. So if there is a real concern ask a manager or even ask the chef themselves if the food that you are going to eat is Paleo or on the Paleo diet.

Tip #14 – CHANGE YOUR SIDE

In many restaurants they will rattle off a whole bunch of side items. If you want the sides ask for a vegetable that is on the Paleo diet. In some cases vegetables may not be listed or an option but it doesn't hurt to ask.

TIP #15 –NO MSG

MSG – Monosodium Glutamate is a flavor enhancer which is added to virtually every pre-packed or processed food item. It has been used for decades and health experts have warned against it for a long time; it is not good for asthma and allergy sufferers and also harms long term health. Bottom line: make sure that you don't get it in your food. Now people usually associate MSG with Asian or Chinese food. This is true but it has also been proven to show up in other places as well i.e. soups, canned food, ready meals, salad dressings and sauces. So if it is a true concern for you just say No to MSG.

TIP #16 – REMOVE TEMPTATIONS

When dining out it is common practice to offer you bread, breadsticks or something along those lines to munch on while you wait. If this is a common practice at the restaurants that you visit just tell the waiter when you are seated not to send any bread or other tempting items to the table. You can always opt for olives to nimble instead.

TIP #17 – CHILL OUT

My final tip is to tell you to chill out. When you go out to restaurants it is a time to relax and enjoy yourself. If for some reason you get something that is not Paleo don't call the code enforcement people or write a nasty letter to headquarters. Eating something that isn't Paleo will not kill you. So just go, eat, drink and be marry for tomorrow is another day. Just don't fall into bad habits OK☐

I home that these tips are helpful when going out on the town and eating with friends and family. Not everything you do will be considered Paleo and that is okay. It is a choice to eat Paleo and not to eat Paleo. If you take Paleo too seriously then it will become an obsession and not a way of life. It is like smoking and drinking you need to know when to do it and when not to do it. Eating Paleo is a lifestyle not a religion. So do the best that you can, enjoy life and everything that life has to offer.

Staying Motivated

Motivation

This is a powerful word and it is something that means something different to different people. When you are motivated you have an end goal in mind. You can see the end results just sitting there taunting you, egging you on. When it comes to motivation many people have different reasons and desires.

My personal motivation in life is to be creative and show my creativity. This is why I write. I don't write for the money. I write because I love to tell stories and to tell people about different things. This is one reason why I wrote this book for you today. Others have motivations when it comes to weight loss. This may be one of the reasons why you are reading this book right now. You are motivated in wanting to learn something new about this subject which you don't know already. Well I hope I delivered something new for you. You may be a mother motivated to lose the extra baby weight from a pregnancy. You may be motivated to lose weight because you were in an accident and have gained more weight than you want. You may be motivated to start gaining adding energy since you feel sluggish and just want to feel better. You may want to rid yourself of annoying allergies and dependence on anti-histamine medication.

Motivation is like having a bag filled with wishes. We all have one it is just a matter of making it come true. But the question becomes how do we stay motivated when we just don't see results.

Well the first thing is to go back to the beginning and reconnect with the reasons you started on the Paleo diet in the first place. Was it to fit into those jeans you wore in high school? Is it to fit into a tux or wedding dress? Is it to feel less bloated? Is it to feel in control of your long term health and not to live in fear of dread diseases? How about being able to run and play with your kids or grandkids in the park?

We all have motivations in life and finding a way to stay true to them is a challenge all in itself. If after reflecting on the reason why you started the Paleo diet in the first place you are still not motivated try looking back at all the effort that you have already done to get to where you are. Going backwards for some people is never an option. If you are looking at going backwards and destroying your success that you have achieved then that may be a powerful motivator to move on or keep going.

"I don't have a reverse gear," said Tony Blair once. Well sometimes that is a bad thing, but going back may not be an option. Once people ditch wheat and gluten, they find that eating it again gives them terrible indigestion, heartburn and a lethargic dizzy feeling. When you quit milk, it can actually taste sour and unpleasant when you have it again. Your body actually changes and wants to stay Paleo.

Get a partner. You know it is always easier to quit when the only one you will disappoint is yourself. If you get a partner to go along on the journey with you then it is easier to stay motivated to continue knowing that you will let the other person down if you quit.

Go into competition with yourself or someone else. This is another great motivational technique. If you chart your progress and try to beat it on a daily or weekly basis you can add a level of personal enjoyment to your motivation. If you are teaming up with someone then you can compete with them on a friendly level. If you go into competition with someone make sure you do it on a friendly basis. You never want to go into competition to hurt someone's feelings or tear them down for their efforts.

Friendly competition is always a healthy thing. It keeps the interest alive as well as puts a little fun and challenge into the overall process.

The bottom line when it comes to motivation is that you need to find reason to be motivated. You need to look at different and creative ways to stay motivated and to motivate others. At the end of the day it is the end results that matter. The journey will be filled with ups and downs Just make those journeys fun and interesting.

Faq

Well I hope that you have enjoyed your journey into the world of Paleo. I have tried to incorporate as much information as I could into this book. As with anything I am sure that I have missed something or could have covered a topic in better detail. No matter what book you read on any topic you won't get all of the answers that you seek. As a final bid to cover as much as I can in this book I am adding this FAQ section. In this section I will try to answer as many of the questions posed by people in regards to Paleo. I am going to try and answer questions that I have not covered yet in the book but if I did cover them I will try to give a little more of a detailed answer.

Once again I want to thank you for coming on this journey with me through the world of Paleo. I hope that it has inspired you to take a deeper look at Paleo and perhaps even give it a try for a week, month or even longer.

Q. HOW DOES THE PALEO DIET WORK?

A. The Paleo diet works the way God, nature or the universe intended us to eat. When you eat Paleo you are eating foods that don't contain artificial ingredients or manmade preservatives in them. 333 generations ago man started walking the Earth and eating its foods. With the limited population at the time there was no need for preservatives and additives like we have today.

Since we were stronger and more fit back those many years ago it is lead us to believe that removing these items from our food will lead us back down that path. With the countless people who have taken the Paleo challenge the theory has proven itself correct which is why the Paleo diet works.

Q. HOW IS PALEO DIFFERENT FROM OTHER DIETS

A. The Paleo diet is different because it is the natural diet. The Paleo diet is not something that was thought up in a lab or by some geeks in college looking to make a million dollars on some new supplement or food additive. When you look at diets today you see that they are all commercialized. Atkins for example is a diet that you see on television all the time. South Beach is another diet that you see in the stores.

When you hear the word "Diet" you are looking at a manmade term that was developed to sell you something. When "diet" is used in Paleo terms it is referring to the ancient term of what one once ate as a diet. Do you see the difference? A diet in the ancient terms was geared to what was eaten not something to help lose weight.

So to thumb it up, Paleo original diet. Not a fad, not a gimmick!

Q. WHAT ARE OTHER HEALTH BENEFITS FOR GOING PALEO?

A. The main causes of disease are the increases or sudden spikes in high blood sugar levels. When eating in the Paleo style you are removing sugar and sugar related items that cause glucose from your body, so the likelihood of getting sick or catching a disease is limited. Now this is not to say going on the Paleo diet will keep you 100% safe from cancer, heart disease, obesity and other illnesses. It all depends on when you went on the diet, how much damage was already done, what genetic factors run in your family and the list goes on and on. However going on the Paleo diet now, can dramatically reduce your risk factors.

Going on the Paleo diet is a bug step in the right direction but it is not a cure all solution. There is no cure all solution for anything in the world. But the sooner you decide to move towards a Paleo inspired diet and way of life the better off you will be in the long run. Don't believe me? Just try it.

Q. WHAT ABOUT MY BONES IF I AM NOT CONSUMING DAIRY PRODUCTS

A. This is a very good question. Well I am going to try to answer this without breaking out my science book and white lab coat. When it comes to calcium there is a balance that needs to be achieved. In most cases you hear doctors and scientists say that you need to take in so much calcium for healthy teeth and bones. Well this may be true to an extent, it is also a ploy from the dairy industry to sell more milk and milk products.

If you look at milk products they pump that stuff with so many hormones and additives it would kill the cow. Not to get off the subject but if you want to hear a good rant about milk watch the HBO special from Lewis Black. He does a milk bit that gets you rolling on the floor.

But anyways, your bone health is dependent on a balance of Acid and Base that is sent to your kidneys. All food that is digested must go through the kidneys to be screened and cleaned of any toxins. This screened material is then turned into either an acid or a base. Remember acids and bases in science class? Well to make this simple when you are on the Paleo diet the foods that you eat produce the correct acids and bases to promote bone health and growth. When you are on a diet that is not Paleo your body produces the acids and bases that cause bone deficiency.

To truly answer this question in detail I would have to do a lot more in technical terms but the simplest answer is this. Paleo diet good for bones. Non-Paleo diet not good for bones that is why you need milk on non-paleo diets.

Wow. I got through that one.

Q. WHY SHOULD I AVOID SALT ON MY FOOD?

A. Adding additional salt to your diet adds to the net acid that the kidneys. As a result the kidneys go and tap into the bones of your body to get the additional nutrients that were lost by adding the salt. When we add salt to our food we are increasing the drain of nutrients to our banes which makes them weaker which in turn results in bone disease and other health problems.

So is it bad to have salt in our diets? No we need salt to live. The human body is made up of salt and water. Taking salt away just makes it worse. Adding more salt to our bodies is just as bad. It is up to you to find the balance.

Q. DOESN'T THE MEAT WE EAT PROMORE HEART DISEASE

A. Like stated before it all comes down to the type of fats and cholesterol we consume. Years ago we believed that saturated fats and cholesterol were the causes of many diseases such as heart disease, diabetes, cancer and many others. But with advancement of modern science and technology we have found this not to be true. It has been discovered that the grains and other foods that break down in to sugars are the cause of most of those problems. The blood sugar in our bodies reacts causing many of these problems. So to answer this question you want to find natural organic, grass fed meats whenever possible since they contain less of the harmful fats, but in general eating these meats is good for you.

Q. WHEN WE WERE KIDS WE WERE TOLD TO EAT OUR GRAINS SINCE THEY WERE A GREAT SOURCE OF FIBER. WHAT ARE YOU TELLING ME, THAT THIS ISN'T TRUE ANYMOE?

A. Well Veronica... wait a minute that was Santa Clause. Well sorry to have to break the bad news to you again. Through recent studies it has been found that a 1,000 calorie serving of fruits and vegetables has two to seven times more grams of fiber than whole grains.

When it comes to fruits and vegetables the fiber contained is considered to be more heart healthy fiber and cholesterol reducing fiber than those found in whole grain. It is funny how things work out sometimes. When we were kids and we added bananas and strawberries to our cereal in the morning, which was better for us than the cereal itself.

Q. CAN I EAT THIS DIET IF I AM A VEGETARIAN

A. YES. IF THEY WANT TO THAT IS.

The problem is, that you have to change your belief as a vegetarian. When you are a vegetarian you don't eat meat. So it is impossible to be on the Paleo diet and not eat meat. Now you can eat seafood which I know vegetarians eat but as far as meat and poultry that has to a decision that is be made by each individual person. So on one side of the coin the Paleo diet can be eaten by anyone who wishes to follow the guidelines which can include vegetarians. On the other hand since eating meat is a critical part of the Paleo diet and vegetarians don't eat those items going Paleo is no no for them.

Most vegetarians I know eat loads of cheese, pastry and pasta. If you want to be a Paleo Vegetarian, you have to go Vegan and also quit wheat, grains and sugar. It is in addition very hard to be a vegan with no legumes, rice or potatoes. To be a Paleo Vegan is a highly specialized diet, which I cannot say I recommend. I have actually done it myself, but I have eaten legumes instead of the meat. It is hard and you have to be a very good cook.

Q. HOW YOUNG CAN SOMEONE START EATING PALEO?

A. Paleo is a lifestyle so it can be started at any age. In fact the sooner you start off on a Paleo diet the better off you will be. I know what you are saying, our kids need milk in school to become big and strong. The problem with that is that there is so many hormones in the milk kids that are only seven and eight look like they are thirteen and fourteen years old. Now I am not a scientist or nor do I claim to be. I am also not a doctor so my medical opinion is moot at this point. But go and do your own observations. Go to your kid's school if you have kids and if you don't have kids drive by an elementary or middle school some time and just look at the kids that are there running and playing. When you are there ask yourself, do these kids look like the kids that were out there playing when you went to school?

I joke sometimes when I see large kids, not fat but tall for their age, walk into to schools. I joke and say, "Well they drink a lot of milk." Now I don't know this for a fact but it is a pretty good assumption. Now from my understanding there is no logical reason why kids should be that big at that age. My only conclusion is it is because of the food that they eat and drink. In my street there are 12 families with children and I have lived here and seen those kids grow up over 17 years – every child, boy or girl is now taller than both their parents.

Look at all the health problems kids are having these days. How many kids do you know that are autistic? Me personally, I know three. Three. How many did you know growing up? If you look at the world today problems like autism, mental problems, behavioral problems, increase in sexual maturity, allergies, asthma and ADD. The list goes on and on.

There has to be a causal factor in this. And the only one I can find is what goes into our food and drink. So if we were to start ourselves and our children on a Paleo diet early in life maybe these conditions would stop and perhaps even reverse themselves. If we get them on a Paleo diet before they have children maybe, just maybe we can stop these issues from hitting yet another generation.

Q, WHAT CAN'T I EAT ON PALEO

A Anything with an artificial ingredients. These ingredients include but are not limited to aspartame, calcium sorbate, monosodium glutamate more commonly known a (MSG), nitrates, potassium bromate, saccharin, sorbic acid, artificial colors and artificial sweeteners.

Fizzy drinks are also something that you can't have on the Paleo diet. Now this is a crusher for many. Soda is not a natural creation plus it contains tons and tons of sugars. So this is out on the Paleo diet. Try mixing apple juice with a squeeze of lemon and sparkling spring water – you can add mint, ginger or any other fruit juice for an exciting, tasty and refreshing drink.

Partially hydrogenated oils are also bad. These oils were created by man not nature. They were created to help keep oil good on the shelves for months and sometimes even years at a time. The problem with these was that they contained what is known as Tran's fats. When this was discovered there was a public outcry to have the companies remove the Trans fats from the shelves. This caused the manufacturers to either become sneaky and reword their labels or go back to the drawing board and come up with another way to produce a longer lasting oil.

Junk Food – now I know that this is a killer.

The main problem is that the caveman didn't have Pepsi or Coke products. They ate what was off the land. They couldn't go and get a snickers to satisfy them or a nice cold soda to refresh their thirst from a long hard day of chasing down their dinner. If they could, I don't think modern man would be where we are today. I think if the caveman had had the foods that we have today the human race would have died out thousands of years ago. You know, I hope that time travel doesn't exist somewhere. If it did we'd all be screwed.

Fast foods – Fast food is another thing you can't have on Paleo.

When it comes to fast food, they are cooked in harmful oils and have many additives, not to mention always containing milk and wheat.

No Grains – This means no bread, no cereal, no crackers or anything else made with grains. Those starting on the Paleo diet swear that cutting grains from their diet made them feel a million times better.

Dairy

Now this is a tricky subject. Since early man wasn't in the habit of domesticating animals, it is not likely that they would have milked them, drank the milk, made dairy products and so on. Now we can be wrong about this fact no one was around to video tape them so the actual truth will never be known but from observation and deductive reasoning it has been concluded that early man did not drink milk or have dairy products.

Processed foods – This is another thing that caveman didn't have. There were no prepackaged bison on a stick or microwavable dino nuggets. The creation of processed food didn't come about until hundreds upon hundreds of years of advancement later. Since processing the food involved adding chemicals and other artificial ingredients eating processed foods is a no on Paleo.

Legumes –

This is another tricky one when it comes to Paleo. Since legumes or beans come from the earth, it is possible that the early caveman ate these as part of their diet. But since the legumes cause inflammation and a slew of other gut problems they are not considered to be an official part of the Paleo diet. So if you do eat them you are not eating true Paleo. If you have legumes from time to time be sure to soak for 24 hours and cook very well to negate some of the negative effects.

Potatoes – These are also not on the Paleo diet list. Why is this? Potatoes grow in the ground and cavemen ate what was in the ground? Well that is why it is a grey area when it comes to Paleo. When growing a potato it takes a lot of cultivating of the land as well as other factors that weren't available to cavemen of that era. Now it is true that they may have stumbled upon a wild form of potato but as far as the modern potato that we know and love, caveman didn't have access to those since it is a totally different process of growing and harvesting.

FINAL WORD ON FAQ

Well I hope that I have answered some of the more popular FAQ's. I am sure again that I could probably sit and write and write about these all day long. In fact I could probably write an entire book answering questions when it comes to Paleo and the Paleo diet.

From this point I will let you go and explore more about Paleo. Take what you have learned here and apply it towards your growing education on this subject. If you have any further questions in regards to Paleo, the Paleo lifestyle and anything else Paleo the Internet is filled with content that you can use to further your education. But from here I will lead you into the conclusion of the book and hope that your journey into the world of Paleo is as fun and exciting as it was for me. Good luck and healthy eating.

Conclusion

Whew, we have been on an amazing journey haven't we? If we take a good hard look at our world and the things in it we will find an amazing balance. When we try to mess with that balance our entire world reacts in a way to try to return to that balance.

This is where the Paleo diet comes in. When you look at the Paleo diet you are looking into our past and the way things were and the way things should be today. Through this journey I hope you have learned more about the world of Paleo and what it can do for you.

When you look at Paleo it is a diet that is not meant to help you lose weight it is a diet that helps you live better. When you go Paleo you are eating what the world had given you in its original natural form. You are eating the fish and seafood from the sea. You are eating the animals from the land and you are consuming the birds from the sky.

It is said we are born from earth and to earth we shall return. This is very true. When we try to deny this universal truth we have problems such as disease and illness.

In this book I have given you a seven day plan to get you started on your road to Paleo. I have also introduced you to ten celebrities that have taken on the Paleo challenge and support it.

We have talked about exercise and why it is so important to maintaining a balance between body and mind. I also have given you many questions that others have asked concerning the Paleo diet with answers and resources to go and follow up on. I have given you tips, tricks and much more that you can use to further your education.

Taking Paleo to heart is one of the best choices that you can possibly take on. I hope that I have convinced you to at least look further into Paleo. If you were to take anything away from this book I would want it to be this. "Try it."

Thank you for going on this journey with me and I hope that you try the Paleo diet.

To your health and to your success.

www.ingramcontent.com/pod-product-compliance
Lightning Source LLC
Chambersburg PA
CBHW071832080526
44589CB00012B/997